MW01482357

★ TAC...
FITNESS (40+)
FOUNDATION
REBUILDING

FOR BEGINNERS OR
RECOVERING FROM INJURY

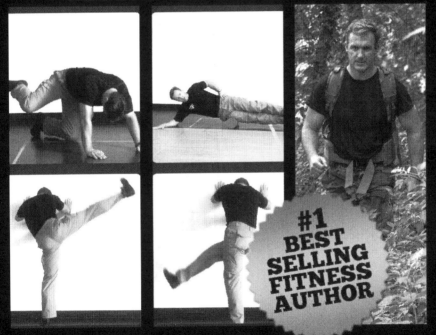

#1
BEST
SELLING
FITNESS
AUTHOR

STEW SMITH, CSCS, USN (SEAL)

ATTENTION:
A Special Note about how this book was created.

Dear Former Athlete Over 40,

Thank you for claiming your copy of "*Tactical Fitness (40+) – Foundation Rebuilding – For Beginners or Recovering from Injury.*"

This book will teach you critical physical rebuilding, recovery and maintenance skills, tools and techniques, and help you rebuild solid habits of fitness that everyday people over 40 need to understand and apply.

This book was originally created as a live interview. Plus, we added exercise pictures, descriptions, links to videos and workouts that focus on all elements of fitness, and allow for proper recovery for the tactical athlete.

That's why Section One <u>reads as a conversation</u> rather than a traditional "book" that talks "at" you. However, Section Two and Section Three are more of the traditional fitness book with exercise and workout descriptions / workout charts.

This interview is with what I call the perfect representative for whom this book is made. I also want you to feel as though I am talking "with" you (the reader), much like a coach or a conversion with a friend AND get a world class workout for someone who needs to get back on the fitness wagon.

I felt that creating the material this way would make it fun for you as we discuss these important topics and put them to use quickly, rather than wading through hundreds of pages of why this book is ideal for you.

Get ready to rebuild your fitness and learn how to use recovery methods to feel better and more invigorated each day. Learning how to train effectively to build a fitness foundation and how to actively pursue recovery is the goal of this book.

PS – if you prefer the PDF version, please email me and I will email you the PDF file as Kindle can sometimes not quite get the charts centered on one page.

Sincerely,

Stew Smith

Table of Contents

Meet Stew Smith

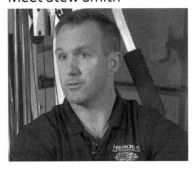

Stew Smith is an expert in Tactical Fitness training, coaching, and writing whose accomplishments include:

Education:

- US Naval Academy Graduate
- Navy SEAL Training Graduate
- Certified Strength and Conditioning Specialist (CSCS)

Work History:

- Trained thousands of Navy Midshipmen at the Naval Academy
- Trained thousands of military, police, spec ops, and firefighters
- 20+ year history of coaching, training, presenting Tactical Fitness

Awards, Titles, and Designations:

- Amazon Best Selling Fitness Author
- Published Author of Tactical Fitness books and training programs (40)
- Created StewSmith.com 1998
- Created StewSmithFitness.com 2012
- Selling Books since 1998 and eBooks since 2002.
- Online Coaching since 1998

Personal / Business Info:

- Former US Navy SEAL Officer
- Guest instructor at Naval Academy Summer Seminar training 2400 USNA candidates each year for over 20 years.
- Spec Ops Team Coach at the US Naval Academy
- Founder of "Heroes of Tomorrow" which trains military, special ops, police, SWAT, and fire fighters candidates for FREE.
- Created Podcast – Tactical Fitness Report with Stew Smith (Youtube, iTunes, GooglePlay).
- Featured on Fight Science – Special Ops "Ice Man"
- Full time fitness writer (Military.com, DotDash.com, TheBalance.com) and many other websites and magazines as a freelance writer.
- Works out and writes about it for a living.

Published Books Written by Stew Smith
Tactical Fitness | Tactical Strength | Tactical Mobility
Warrior Workouts – Volume 1
The Complete Guide to Navy SEAL Fitness
Navy SEAL Weight Training Workout
Maximum Fitness
The SWAT Workout
The Special Operations Workout

General Fitness and Nutritional Guides for Everyone
The Beginner / Intermediate Guide to Fitness
Reclaim Your Life - Erin O'Neill Story (beginner / intermediate)
Veterans Fitness - Baby Boomer and a Flat Stomach!
Circuit Training 101 – Beginner / Intermediate Guide to the Gym
The Busy Executive Workout Routine
The Obstacle Course Workout – Prep for Races or Mil, LE, FF
TRX / Military Style Workouts – Adding TRX to Military Prep Workouts

The Military / Special Ops Physical Fitness Workouts
Advanced Maintenance / Recovery Plan
The Combat Conditioning Workout
Air Force PJ / CCT Workout
The UBRR – Upper Body Round Robin Workout / Spec Ops version
Navy SEAL Workout Phase 1
Navy SEAL Workout Phase 2 - 3
Navy SEAL Workout Phase 4 Grinder PT
Navy SWCC Workout
Army Special Forces / Ranger Workout
Army Air Assault School Workout
Army Airborne Workout
USMC RECON Workout
USMC OCS / TBS Workout
USMC IST and PFT
The Coast Guard Rescue Swimmer / Navy SAR Workout
The Service Academy Workout (West Point, Navy, Air Force Academy)
The Navy, Air Force, Marine Corp Boot Camp Workout
The Army OCS and PFT Workout
Military, Police, Fire Fighter PT Test Survival Guide

The Law Enforcement Physical Fitness Workouts
The FBI Academy Workout | FBI Workout Vol 2
The DEA Workout
The FLETC Workout - Ace the PEB
The PFT Bible: Pushups, Sit-ups, 1.5 Mile Run
The Fire Fighter Workout

Contact Stew Smith (Email, mail)

As part of the downloadable, you do have access to email me at any time and I will answer your questions as soon as possible. Below are the ways to contact me for any of the products and services at www.stewsmith.com.

Mail and email addresses:
StewSmith.com
PO Box 122
Severna Park MD 21146
Email - stew@stewsmith.com

Social Media:

Youtube.com : www.youtube.com/stew50smith (podcasts, swim videos)

Facebook: www.facebook.com/stewsmithfitness (Articles / Q & A)

Instagram: www.instagram.com/stewsmith50 (Cool pics, Motivation)

Twitter: www.twitter.com/stewsmith (Articles, Motivation)

FREE Videos in this Book

In this product, there are free downloadable videos and links to nutrition charts, lower back exercises, and more - many demonstrate exercises and show techniques in motion by clicking the hyperlinks in the program. These are also on www.youtube.com/stew50smith

As with any generic fitness program, this may not be right for you and you should adjust accordingly if needed. Consulting a physician is recommended before undertaking any new fitness program.

Tactical Fitness Is For Everyone

Tactical Fitness is a relatively new genre of fitness that is primarily designed for people in the military, and police and fire fighter professions where life or death situations occur as part of the job, and fitness can be the determining factor of surviving. However, Tactical Fitness can be for everyone. Consider Tactical Fitness as Functional Fitness for regular LIFE, as well as life or death situations.

If you notice, during emergencies or natural disasters, there are two types of people: Those who need saving and rescuing, and those capable of helping.

We all should have a certain level of tactical / practical fitness that could help us save our own lives or the lives of our loved ones in the event of a disaster (natural or man-made). Of course, basic health and wellness cannot be overlooked either. The goal of this book is to help people with the roadmap to being able to save themselves or others in potentially dangerous situations, as well as build healthy habits for the rest of their long lives.

The Tactical Fitness 40+ is a three-phase program (this is phase 1):

Phase 1 – *Tactical Fitness 40+ Foundation Rebuilding*

Phase 2 – *Tactical Fitness 40+ Taking It To The Next Level*

Phase 3 – *Tactical Fitness 40+ Ready to Compete*

And the capstone of the series: <u>Tactical Fitness for the Athlete Over 40: Actively Pursuing Recovery and Healthy Maintenance</u>. The overwhelming positive reaction to this initial advanced program prompted the need for a better progression. Now, the progression is broken up into three phases so the entire spectrum of fitness levels can have a program to rebuild, maintain, and increase physical activity and longevity.

We show you the evolution of the process to go from a low level of fitness and health, to rebuilding the fitness foundation focusing on all the elements of fitness: flexibility, mobility, endurance, stamina, strength, power, speed and agility. We do this very slowly and progressively with over a year's worth of training in the four programs.

The next section is an interview with a gentleman feeling the struggle of age, health and wellness, mental toughness, and physical performance. We all have these issues at some point.

Chapter One: Stew Smith and the Fitness Foundation

Stew Smith:	[To the reader] Thank you for getting this ebook or book. If you prefer the PDF version of the book and you ordered the printed version or the Kindle, please let me know and I will email it to you, as the PDF tends to be better for the exercise charts in this book.

This is a project I've been working on for a while, focusing on the aging athlete. Even though you may not consider yourself "an athlete," I am going to explain how you really are. We are all Tactical Athletes. Because I spent most of my professional writing life creating programs for the 18 to 20-year-old to prepare themselves in tactical fitness for military, law enforcement, firefighting professions, I started this 20 years ago. And many of my readers that I started writing for back then are now 38 - 40 years old and still in the game. Many have a long history of injuries, and aches and pains that they are trying to fight through, so they can still be active. Many are having to start all over again at beginning levels due to a variety of reasons, from illness, injuries, or burnout after 15+ years of war.

This program is for the person who needs to build or rebuild their fitness foundation. I want to introduce you to Gerald Poole. The reason I brought Gerald on here is because I think he personifies who I am trying to write for.

There is a segment of the population that I have neglected in my writings. And that's why this whole series is built on people like Gerald. *This is the program for 35, 45, 50-year-olds, whether you are civilian, former military, police, or fire service or still active.* Whether you are broken and are trying to rebuild, or have been seriously ill and trying to rebuild, or haven't done anything for 20 years and just need to get started again building your fitness foundation. If this is your story, this is your program. |
| Stewart Smith: | Gerald has had a unique history of this process, and without me talking about it, let's hear it from him. So, |

Gerald, welcome. First of all, Gerald thank you for doing this project with me. I think it's really cool that you are going to help me verbalize some issues that are definitely hard to write about. So, let's hear about you. Tell us about your background, your experience in life that's led you to your current position, as well as past fitness histories.

Gerald Poole:

I don't have a tremendously intense background when it comes to sports. I would say that I've always been an active person. In high school, I was a tennis player, and actually a musician for a lot of my high school and college days. I would say physically I was really active on the tennis court, and then also in the weight room. I did a lot of weightlifting, but typical bodybuilding type of training three times a week and then alternating three times a week with cardio workouts. Now, I'm 43. So, when I talk about high school and I talk about college, you can kind of figure out how long ago that may have been. I was never too intense with any one physical activity. When I talk about the bodybuilding workouts, those types of workouts, at least in my opinion, are obviously good for you. Lifting weights, building muscle, getting leaner, increasing bone density, and increasing your cardio are all great. But it was mostly done for *aesthetics*, especially when I was younger. Everyone wants to get bigger muscles and things like that. That was my true foundation.

Stewart Smith:

Okay. So, you have a decent fitness foundation. What would you say about your friends? Your workout partners, your teammates? How are they doing in comparison to you? Along this journey, you maybe had workout partners, or you have friends and mentors that you've met along your fitness journey.

Gerald Poole:

That has changed over the years. Now, what I'm looking for is functionality, and being capable of doing things because I am fit. And when you talk about where are some of my friends, and some of the events I've done, transitioning from that bodybuilding aesthetics kind of mindset to more functionality and capability ... I went from training for aesthetics to saying, "How can I get tougher? How can I be someone who isn't going to quit when things get hard? How can I become somebody that really trains hard, and then goes, okay, well, this was a nice 40-minute workout, but how can I handle four more hours?"

So, when you ask about the people that I've been hanging out with, I came to believe that to be an important part of becoming more mentally tough, and just better at endurance events. Surrounding myself with like-minded people was important, even though it's hard to find people like that in your immediate circle of friends. That mindset is not as common as you would hope it to be. So, I started turning to online sources for learning how to think that way. And a lot of that had to do with watching your videos, or other Navy SEAL videos, reading about GoRuck stories, and certain books by special operators, and things like that.

So, I really went from hanging out with people who wanted to get big in the gym to people seeking something different out of their training.

Stewart Smith:	Oh, yeah. I know exactly what you are talking about, but you know what? I think many people are lying if they don't say that was probably what got them in the weight room in the first place.
Stewart Smith:	I was 14 years old. I remember that all the time. It was a contest. How much you could bench. When I was growing up, it was Joe Weider workout books, in the 80s. Three sets of eight, and do a couple of exercises, and I thought I was done with a workout.
	But yeah. Things evolve, and things change along with your goals and with your desire. So, what is your goal now? Let's talk about a short-term goal of one to two years, and then let's talk about a long-term goal of 50 plus.
Gerald Poole:	I think I'll start by saying ... For me, this became the journey to becoming more mentally tough. And why is that important? Why did I want to do that? What significance did it have for me?

In my early 30s, I was thinking, "I've got to be capable of doing more." I want to be able to look back on things that I've done, whether it was last week, or 20 years ago, or whatever, and say, "I did really hard things, and I hung in there." And I want to become my best self. I want to know when things got hard, I didn't quit.

And I hate to say this, but I've got to be honest. I started getting interested in reading about Navy SEALs. And there are some Navy SEAL camps, and military-inspired events out there. And I thought, "How cool would it be to do these events?" And I failed.

Stewart Smith: You know, they are good gut checks.

Gerald Poole: I failed...

Stewart Smith: They are really tough gut checks. You are talking about Mark Divine's program right?

Gerald Poole: Yes.

Stewart Smith: Great guy. Great gut check. Great challenge.

Gerald Poole: Yeah. Great challenge. And as embarrassing as it is to talk about, it's very real. I think you need to talk about what's real in order to get better. I do not want to sugar-coat things and make excuses for why things didn't work. I have to be honest with myself.

Stewart Smith: But before you do, though, let's talk about this. Your foundation was gym workouts, aesthetics, maybe 30, 45-minute workouts. Something longer?

Gerald Poole: Yes.

Stewart Smith: And then you say, "Alright, I'm going to do this. I'm going to start focusing on these tougher events as mental toughness challenges." And so that's where I talk a lot about tactical fitness. And it really does depend on your fitness foundation before you start attempting some of these hard challenges. The transition from this fitness foundation of power lifting or weightlifting or other sports into these harder challenges may take a good year or more. This is what I tell tactical athletes that are trying to be military, law enforcement, and firefighters.

However, the reason you are being interviewed here is because you are my tactical athlete, personified, for civilian purposes. And what I mean by that is ... We all need to be tactical athletes. And maybe we call them "functional athletes," or "functional fitness," or whatever. There's so many terms to describe what I'm trying to say. But, basically, it is this: When there's an accident that happens, there are two types of people. There are people that need to be saved, and there are people who are doing the saving.

Gerald Poole: Right.

Stewart Smith: And I have been a big proponent of being in a good fitness foundation and abilities so that when something happens, I can be the helper. So, when something goes down, I want to be able to be the guy who can save my family, save a victim from whatever circumstance, or myself for that matter. Having the confidence that my physical ability can save lives is a huge mental boost that not many people have. The lack of this confidence can detour people from accepting new challenges and bettering themselves as well. It spills over into other areas of your life too.

Gerald Poole: Right.

Chapter Three: Moving Passed Failure – Developing Tactical Fitness

Stewart Smith: When we talk about tactical fitness, I want people to realize that it's not just for military, law enforcement, or firefighters. ***It's really for everybody.*** And I wanted to share that with you, because after talking with you for a while, I realized this is what you were trying to do.

Gerald Poole: One hundred percent. And that's exactly right. I don't want to be just a muscle head. I want to be someone who can be capable when something happens. Because today, I think it is very relevant.

Unfortunately, you turn on the news, and you see crazy things happen every day, either natural or man-made. Or what if my kid falls into a swimming pool? Am I going to be able to jump in there and get him without getting into trouble myself? But I think being a tactical athlete is more relevant to civilians than most civilians even believe, or would begin to imagine. I think it's very relevant.

And it doesn't have to be catastrophic events. It doesn't have to be me trying to save my children and my wife from tragedy, or getting the kids out of the house in a fire. I have a two-year-old and a five-year-old. It can be just both of them wanting to be carried at the same time and being able to do that.

Stewart Smith: Yeah. There you go.

Gerald Poole: And that happens a lot, I am always carrying them. And you talk about aging athletes ... At 43 and well into my 50's and 60's," I want to be rolling with them still.

Stewart Smith: Yeah. That's a good one.

Gerald Poole: And I think the tactical mindset and being a tactical athlete will enable me to do that.

Stewart Smith: Absolutely. What about some of the things you have done? Whenever you started on this journey with these tactical fitness challenges, what were some of the events that you did? What made you re-circle and come about attacking these in a different way?

Gerald Poole: So, that's really, for me, the crux of this. We mentioned SEALFIT, and Mark Divine's camps early on. And again, being honest with myself is hard. But I think you have to be honest in order to get better, and you have to realize the strength in saying, "Hey,

I can't be satisfied with failing. I need to confront what I did wrong, and I need to figure out how to fix it, and I need to move forward."

So, when I was in my early 30s and I wanted to try some of these things, like SEALFIT, I still had that mentality of the bodybuilding type workouts. I was thinking, "Hey, wouldn't it be cool to go through this? Wouldn't it be cool to do that? Wouldn't it be cool to tell somebody that I did this?" ***And those are not the right reasons to do it.*** That's garbage, to be able to go, "Oh, I want to do this so I can tell someone I did it." And I tried to do the SEALFIT camp, initially, doing bodybuilding workouts three times a week, and cardio three times a week for 40 minutes or an hour. And then having the mentality of, "Oh, this would be cool. I can say that I did this." I failed miserably. It was bad. I quit. I just quit.

Stewart Smith:	I tell people all the time, man ... There's no 30, 40-minute workout that's going to prepare you for a day of Spec-Ops training and I think that was your first issue. But, you really do have to put in your time to training like this. When you say you failed, what happened? Was it a physical breakdown? Was it being cold, being wet and miserable? Mentally challenging? When you say you failed, what happened?
Gerald Poole:	Great questions. Because, admittingly, I quit twice. And both for very different reasons. The first reason was I just had no clue what I was getting into. I had no clue at all. I was under-prepared from a physical and a mental standpoint. I just had no idea. And I had no idea about the intensity, about the pacing. I had no idea about the types of exercises. I thought a plank hold for any more than 30 seconds was impossible and that people did not do such things.

I just was not prepared at all. And I think I made it through about six hours. A lot of it was mental, and I just didn't understand that at the time.

A year came and went, and I realized there was a big lack of maturity, emotional awareness and emotional intelligence. And I kind of mix all that stuff in with mental toughness. I think maturity and emotional intelligence are critical in developing your mental toughness. Then I went back a second time and just quit right before I even started. And that was for a different reason. Mainly anxiety.

I've had a hard time controlling fear in my life. And I would have all these ideas in my head about what I wanted to accomplish, or what I wanted to achieve. And it seemed so clear. And I would go to execute, and it would just fall apart because of that anxiety.

But the second time around, all of these Crossfit guys were there, some of the best Crossfit guys in the world. I showed up there, and I'm like, **"I'm not going to be able to hang with these guys. This is modeled after Hell Week. It's modeled after being a good team member, about pulling your weight, about helping your team. I'm not going to be able to help these guys. I'm going to be a liability."** So, right off the bat, that type of thinking got into my head, and I just was like, "**Don't even try to hang with these guys.**"

Stewart Smith: That is when you have to stop listening to yourself and start TALKING to yourself – just positively.

Gerald Poole: And so those are really two different reasons at two different attempts of why I tried and I quit. And so this was in my early 30s. I'm 43, now. And I kind of resigned to the fact that, "**This isn't for you.**" However, we talk about having powerful WHYS and I have a totally different set of WHYS now.

So those ideas went dormant for several years, and then in started getting that itch again in my late 30s. And the reason why is because I got married, and I had kids. And my WHYS for what kind of Dad I wanted to be shaped why I started getting back into this and saying, "No, no, no, you **_CAN_** do this. You just have to take a different approach."

Stewart Smith: There you go. Yeah. You know what? WHYS, they come in all different sized packages. Some people's

"WHY" is just because they like the adrenaline rush. For some it's, *"I want to do it because I can show people I can do it, and show them they are wrong for doubting me".* There is no good or bad why, I think.

But what you went through, there is a huge roadblock that I think many people today have. Most people probably wouldn't even consider attempting what you've done, or what you tried to do. But I think there is a very big group that are in that zone of, *"I'd like to do that, but I'm not sure how I could prepare for it. I'm not sure if I'm capable of doing that."*

But I will say this, and I tell this to everybody, is that your body is ten times stronger than your mind will ever let it be, if that makes sense.

Gerald Poole: Absolutely. Yes.

Stewart Smith: If you can disengage that little part of your brain, especially the anxiety before an event, the pain of going through the event, all those little things that make us say we want to stop, you will one day realize that your body is ten times stronger than your mind will let it be. And you have to think about this, our brain is built to keep our body alive, and survive. These are natural survival thoughts, and techniques, and skills that your brain has come up with through the eons to keep you alive. Your brain saying, "No, you better not do this, that's stupid," is there to keep you alive.

Gerald Poole: Right.

Stewart Smith: It's unbelievable what your body can do. So, what I try to do, and I think what a lot of these programs try to do, is try to tap into that part of the brain that is going to give you some unbelievable abilities, physically, but also some confidence into handling anything that comes your way in the future. Whether that is having to stay up all night to get a job done, whatever that task is, it is amazing what some of these programs do for you. And I admire you for trying it, and I admire you for turning around and trying it again.

You got through this roadblock. What's next for you?

Gerald Poole:

Yeah. So, good commentary on that, because I think you hit on something just now, but also I think you've talked about this in your podcast, and it is that whole idea of mental toughness. I became obsessed with it. What does it mean? This elusive concept of being mentally tough. And you watch videos of Special Ops guys, or others, and you say, "That's something that I will never be able to possess." Or, "That's something that I can't understand." And I think that, while I'll never be an Olympic athlete, for example, I think we sell ourselves short with how much potential we have with "**becoming mentally tough.**"

I think it boils down to—at least for me—some people might just get it right off the bat and be super mentally tough, and not have to go through this process. But for me it was being exposed to difficult things incrementally, and having little victories. I think you mentioned that in one of your podcasts. "Finding the fuel when the tank is empty or getting comfortable being uncomfortable." Both are so true when trying to define mental toughness.

it started with me going, "**Look. I have two kids that I want to not just take care of as babies and children, but I want to raise them to be certain kinds of adults.**" And I want them to be kind people. I want them to be capable people. I want them to be adjusted. I want them to be strong. Because, there's a lot of fragile people out there, and I **_don't_** want to be one of them. I don't want either of my kids to be one. I don't want, when something gets hard, for them to go, "**Oh, I can't do it," or, "I'm going to quit." Because life is going to be full of that stuff.**

Stew, I started believing, "**I've got to go back and finish these things I started,**" because I can't teach them to do that if I don't do the same thing. I can't teach them to never quit if I've been a quitter. I can't teach them to do difficult things if I don't do difficult things.

We talk about these military-inspired events. I looked into doing a GORUCK. I started with a GORUCK Light. Three or four years ago. And I wasn't in the right kind of shape, or the shape I'm in now, or the shape I will be two years from now. But that gave me that taste of, "*All right. Let's do something challenging on a smaller scale*." That's a short-term, smaller goal that I can achieve, get that patch, and say, "*Okay. I can start building my way up to these more difficult events*."

And the most recent event I did that I'm pretty proud of was the GORUCK Mogadishu Mile – a 24 hour Heavy, a 12 hour Tough, and a 6 hour Light together. All back to back to back over a weekend. I think I slept for an hour, maybe. It was tough.

Stewart Smith: Damn. That's awesome. GORUCK, by the way - I have to give a plug to GORUCK, because they do such a great job, not only with their great backpacks, but their events. Their events are really life changing for people.

Gerald Poole: Absolutely. Aside from doing a 5K or a Turkey Fun Run or something like that, this gives you the opportunity to start pushing yourself. The Lights are shorter. They're not necessarily easier. But you put on your rucksack, you have to carry a certain amount of weight in it, and you travel a certain distance with a team carrying heavy things and doing PT along the way.

Stewart Smith: Getting comfortable being uncomfortable one step at a time.

Gerald Poole: Yes. And it's something I think about a lot. So, in any case, I finished this super-long event. Some of the people there could run circles around me doing PT. And one of these guys was just amazing. He was over 50. You see all these people coming together of varying ages and backgrounds, and you think, "*These are NOW my people and workout partners and motivational friends."* They get it and these events started giving me goals and things to look forward to, which also generated an amazing amount of happiness for me.

The biggest take away for me was, "*I can do things that are difficult."* I would've failed this GORUCK if I didn't start incrementally and build myself up to it. And so, now I want to get to the point where I can go back to Mark Divine's camp and get through it. And that's one of my long-term goals. And there's a couple of other things I want to try, as well.

Stewart Smith: Nice.

Gerald Poole: This last event was six weeks ago, and I lost toenails, had blisters and it hurt. And just taking steps became excruciating. And it was one of those things where I thought, "**Don't quit, because this event will be over. Your feet will heal. But if you quit, you're never going to be able to redeem yourself from that.**" And so, as painful as it was, I kept moving. And when I was finished with that, I was changed.

Stewart Smith: Nice. I think, in there, somewhere, you discovered - what mental toughness is. There's a hard-to-find definition. Some people will say, *"You want mental toughness? Just start getting tougher." Which is great. That's a great, simplistic way of looking at it. But there's some mystery behind it, too, such as "Finding the fuel when the tank is empty.*" I think that is a unique definition for what mental toughness is. And it is pure heart and will. You willed yourself to be able to do that.

Gerald Poole: Absolutely. And I think I overcomplicated it. I overcomplicated it for years. It was not in some motivational quote. It's not some complicated recipe. It's getting comfortable being uncomfortable in increments increasingly more difficult each time, and building on that thought of, "**Hey, I stuck with this. Next time I'm going to make it more difficult.**" Next time, I did it. Made it more difficult. I stuck with it.

Stewart Smith:	And that's no joke, man. Let me just tell you something. That Mogadishu mile, that is very similar to the exact same type of training we put our candidates through to prepare them for SEAL training. Because there's a little thing they used to call Mini-BUDS, that you would go through. And it's basically a 36-hour Heck Day. So instead of a 120-hour Hell Week that you're going to endure at your fourth week of SEAL training, it's a 36-hour version of that.
	And people come to terms with a lot of things. ***"Do I really want to do this in my future?"*** And many people come back or do not. And then they have to progress a little more to find their weaknesses in these things.
	And I think that's where you're starting to see your success. You've acknowledged some weaknesses. You've addressed them. You've tested them through these challenges, and now those weaknesses aren't so much weaknesses anymore. They are now borderline strengths. Because we all come to the table with certain strengths and weaknesses. And I think, it is mainly through honesty and maturity that you have to realize this to move forward.
Gerald Poole:	Absolutely.
Stewart Smith:	I think you're doing that. I love your term, you were "overcomplicating things."
Gerald Poole:	I think people sell themselves short and they overcomplicate it. It's just doing it. But it's acknowledging where you are. If you're a guy reading this right now that's a collegiate wrestler, you're way beyond what I can do. But if you're someone who's never exercised before, and you're 20 pounds overweight, and you're sitting on the couch, and you think, "***Geez, it would be cool to do something like that and challenge myself, but I couldn't do it,"*** you're mistaken. You can do it. It's just that you have to start incrementally, and you

have to build upon each tiny little victory until you say, ***"Okay, I'm going to set that goal to do a GORUCK Light in six months."*** Or whatever it is.

Stewart Smith: And the journey's different for everybody.

Gerald Poole: Exactly.

Stewart Smith: The journey to get there is going to be different for everybody, with your logical progressions to prepare for these type of events.

Gerald Poole: Many don't realize that. I think. At least, I didn't, because I thought, "Well, if I'm not mentally tough right off the bat, if I can't go finish this camp, then it's just not for me." That's wrong.

Stewart Smith: Yes. In fact, in a military term, these events are called "***stress inoculations.***" And they start off with you getting up out of bed, early, before work, when you are probably at your most comfortable you will ever be in a day. Let's face it, there's nothing more comfortable than being on a pillow with covers over you, and laying down in bed. And then you hear that alarm go off at 4:30, or 5:30 in the morning, and that is a very uncomfortable feeling. The comfortable version is to go push that snooze button, or turn the alarm off, and just stay in bed for longer.

The uncomfortable version is getting up and making that a habit. And then, that is kind of the beginning of this stress inoculation. The next step is getting out of the house and going for a run. Or jumping in a swimming pool. It's never warm when you do that, first thing in the morning. That's probably one of the hardest things for me. I dip my toe in the pool and say "***This is going to suck.***" But you jump in anyway. It takes about a hundred meters for the cold to wear off, and you're in it.

All these little things are just little stress inoculations that, like you were saying, "It is building you to be a more mentally tough, resilient person." To be able to handle any future stress that comes about.

Stewart Smith:	And another thing, too, you mentioned - seeing that 50-year-old guy in there kicking butt. That has always motivated me. When I see guys older than me doing it, and getting it done, I say, **"All right. I like this. This is really good."** Because I think there are a lot of benefits to seeing something in order for you to believe it's true. There's a saying. "**You have to see it to believe it**."
Gerald Poole:	Right.
Stewart Smith:	And when you can see people finishing these events, you can say, "I can do that. He's 20 years older than me. I should be able to do that."
	There are training programs that can get you to that level – this is one of many I have created. They work if you do them. This is all about learning. I think some humility in there is very key. It's always good to keep learning. These are processes to get you to that next level. I am still learning everyday and trying out new programs.
Gerald Poole:	The humility part - Get rid of the ego. That was such a big deal for me. Yes, I know, I failed. I quit. I quit twice. I have to acknowledge that and say, "It's okay, because I'm turning things around. I'm going back to finish what I started," or **"I'm learning how not to quit**." And I couldn't have got to this place unless I had gone through that. Unless I had gone through the failures and the quitting, and the desire to get back up there and finish some of these things.
	So, I think ego can be a big, big roadblock to achieving things. And I think it's important to make sure that you remove that, and you start from wherever you are. Treat yourself like a beginner – like you say. You don't have to be happy with where you are, but you can be content with going, "Okay, I have to start at some place. And I can't be an excellent athlete until I'm an intermediate athlete."
	But one more thing that you were talking about when you mentioned the programs you were writing. So, I've tried a bunch of different programs. And a lot of

them, if not all of them, are military based, predominantly Special Operations, SEAL-based training regimens. And there's a lot of great ones out there.

For me, that was the problem, that there are so many sources. However, the reason why I gravitated towards you is because the programming became specific to me as a person. I wasn't getting a prefab email of, "**Here. Here's what you need to do today**." Which ... and again, a lot of these programs are amazing, but what's unique about yours is that the programming's specific to the individual.

And so that's why I gravitated towards you. Because you make the training regimen for me each week, and not only is it specific to what I did last week, it's specific to my individual goals. But it's also tailored to my age. It's tailored to whatever injuries I may be dealing with or trying to prevent, and you take the time to say, "**Hey, look, we have to talk at least each weekend, so each week when I make your program, I can make sure that it's a logical progression from what you did last time**."

Stewart Smith: Yes. That is what we do. And it does work. I've been doing it for almost 20 years - long before people really thought there was an internet business. But, like I said, I find that your story, where you have come from, and where you are now, and where you want to go, is ideal for you taking it to the next level. Because you had a foundation coming in, and you've built upon that foundation. And now it's time for you to move on from the aches and pains of previous challenges, and build upon, and ... Let's take it to the next level.

So, for me, especially for the guy over 40, and myself, too, periodization programming has been a lifesaver. And the way I have arranged these workouts throughout the year to progressively work through ALL the elements of fitness: strength, power, muscle stamina, endurance, speed and agility, and mobility and flexibility. You're in a cycle right now where, I think, we're trying to just build more work capacity. We're kind of pushing some of the longer workouts, working on some endurance. But, there's going to be a time when we need to pull back from that, and work on some strength training. Work on some foundation training. Foundation of strength. And that's going to help you be able to endure some of the harder elements in future events that you do.

And that's the periodization programming that I've been doing for 20 years, and I really think it's saved my life. And then the other thing that has saved me has been after 40 years old, I started adding in a mobility day once a week. And that is kind of the key to this program, as well. I'm making this program to rebuild the foundation, and even taking it to the next level. And then the third phase of this program is going to be, "***I'm ready to compete, and go after it.***"

Gerald Poole:

You have to have that. And that's what I like about working with you, is that it could be even mid-week, and I say, "***I think I need a mobility day.***" And we rearrange. Also, one of the best things I have learned is getting in the pool in chest-deep water and doing some of these dynamic stretches. I'd never heard of that before and I didn't know how valuable it would be. You also talk about foam rolling and stretching, too. But getting into the water, into the chest-deep water, and doing some of these dynamic stretches has been the biggest thing that I've done to help me recover that I hadn't been doing before.

Stewart Smith:

Oh, it has saved me. Like I said, I've been doing it now for almost eight years. And I just started writing about it about four years ago. Just because I wanted to really make sure it was working. I always test things out for a couple of years before I write about it. And that's with any workout that I do. But this one, I had to share. And now I'm putting it in all workouts, even for the 22-year-old guy who probably doesn't even need it, typically. But doing it anyway, just because I've seen performance gains on that following two or three workouts after that he typically didn't have, because he didn't take this little "active rest" day.

Because here's what happens. If you put a mobility day in the middle of your week. Let's say you hit it hard Monday, Tuesday. And you have a Wednesday mobility day. Well, normally, that would've been a hard Wednesday workout, and then a hard Thursday workout, a hard Friday workout. And by Friday and Saturday, your workouts are just horrible. You have no juice left, and you're really getting by on fumes. And I've seen a big change, not only in myself, as the aging athlete, but my younger athletes who take this middle mobility day to help with killer performances on Friday and Saturday, which they were lacking before.

Gerald Poole: Right. And they end their week on a high note with that amazing workout, because they had that opportunity to have an active recovery, if you will. Or mobility, or whatever you want to call it, during the week. But that's also key for injuries, too, because, I have three herniated discs. I have a torn disc. I have bone spurs. My lumbar area is a mess. And I have to work with that. I figured out a way to work with it, and these mobility days help me do that. I think they not only help give my body that active recovery that I need, but they also kind of help with some of these injuries that I'm dealing with, as well, and make some of the other harder workouts possible.

Stewart Smith: Yeah. I love it. So, let's just change topic a little bit, and just talk about recovery and maintenance a little more. Is your life stressful? How would you describe your life? You have a normal, stressful life? Do you have stress in your life?

Gerald Poole: Yes. Absolutely. I've worked really hard at being better at dealing with anxiety and it has made me more powerful. I know that sounds weird. But in my own mind, if you can harness some of those things, and overcome them ... So yes - the initial stress of being an anxious person, and then I have a career, and I have two very young kids.

My wife works full time. I work full time. I've been doing jiu-jitsu for a long time. And I want to get to jiu-jitsu a couple times a week, and trying to fit that in. I also try to fit in all these workouts, trying to get up, trying to get the kids to school, trying to make sure they get to bed, trying to make sure they get their teeth brushed. I mean everything!

It would be easy to say, *"I don't have time."* I've heard people say that, and I get it, but then you'll hear people say, "**Well, you need to make time.**" And it's just that simple.

Stewart Smith: Yes. I love it. So, obviously, everybody's life is stressful. I asked that in a joking manner. But you are relieving your stress through these activities, now.

Gerald Poole: Aside from being a father, and enjoying my family, I would say this is more than a hobby to me. I don't want to cheapen it by calling it a "*hobby*," because it's more than that. But it is, aside from being a father, it's the single biggest source of happiness for me, knowing that I'm training. Knowing that I've failed all these things, and I didn't achieve these things, and I decided that wasn't acceptable. I did not give up! Now, I'm going to go back and fix that." That brings me a tremendous source of, not just stress relief, but general happiness. Which, in itself, is stress relief – just being happy.

Stewart Smith: Very good point. So, here's another thing, too. When your life is stressful, and all of ours are. There's no getting around that. Sometimes the last thing you ever want to do on that very stressful day is to do a butt-kicking workout that's going to stress you out even more, physically. But after a very stressful day, doing something challenging for 15, 20 minutes is great. It's a great way to get these fight/flight hormones out of your body. It will help metabolize them through some activity.

Then, you go through a nice, steady, relaxing breathing cycle. It could be as gentle as a walk. It could be a nice, easy jog, low impact cardio, to get the parasympathetic nervous system going again, and just breathing through it. Because deep breathing, meditation, easy cardio, getting more oxygen into your body is a great way to metabolize stress hormones.

I think that's where a lot of people go wrong, is they either do one of two things. They either don't do anything, which is bad, or they just crush it in the weight room, and just adding stress to your central nervous system on top of all this daily stress that we're putting into our lives. And it's harder to recover from that.

Stewart Smith: Once again, there's always a tangible aspect to training. But then there are intangible aspects to training that are very difficult to get to unless you put in the time.

Gerald Poole: That's right. If mental toughness has a lot to do with flexing that mental muscle, and building the mental muscle, then some of the only times that you can do that is when you're doing something like a tough workout or doing things because you did not want to do them. I remember, specifically, when I work out I think about reporting back to you. I think about not quitting, and feeling good about that. But one of the most important things is I know that when I'm halfway through this workout, and I still have a long way to go, and I'm weak, and I'm not feeling like I want to do it, I know that that's a critical time for me to practice flexing the mental muscle. Because when I'm doing a 40-minute workout, or everything's feeling good, I'm not really practicing it. Because it isn't tough.

Stewart Smith: Absolutely. I would say one of my biggest jobs training young people who want to go into these professions, especially the Special Ops professions, is not coming up with great workouts that build them and prepare them for what their future task is. That is one task I need to do. However, I think the biggest thing that I do is I pull the reins on them and say, "No, you don't need to do that." And say, "Why don't you take a recovery day today," instead of preparing for a 50-mile racing event. "Let's pull back."

Gerald Poole:	Right.

Stewart Smith: Because ... I have seen it happen way too many times. Guys that are hard chargers push, and push, and push, and push, and then something breaks. In fact, that's why I even wrote the first Tactical Fitness For the Athlete Over 40 book was because of that. And it's my own story. My own story was me breaking down at age 28 after year, and year, and year of training ridiculously hard. However, this success came with a price. In the end, that success bit me. So now, I teach people that you need to learn how to start training for longevity. And being smart about your stress that you're accumulating every day.

Gerald Poole: Right. And that has a lot to do with removing that ego.

Stewart Smith: Yes.

Gerald Poole: And it's especially difficult for me, Stew, because I'm someone who's trying to come back from failures. And when you're trying to come back from failures, and you're dedicated or motivated to do it, you want to make sure that you're not quitting. And it's really hard to, sometimes, differentiate between "**You need a mobility day, you need a rest day**," and, "**No, you got to get out there and get it done. Even if you have to crawl through it, you have to get it done.**"

I have to learn how to take a day that wasn't programmed in there and make it a mobility day.

Stewart Smith: Yes. Absolutely. I think we all do. I would say that every week I try to do a mobility day. There may be a week, one week out of the month, where I skip it and move on. And that's okay, if you want to do it. But then I make sure the next week I don't skip it. And some weeks, we will do this really hard weekend workout. And I make sure when we come back on Monday, we do a mobility day. And then we get a couple good workouts in, and on Friday, we do another mobility day. So, sometimes there are actually times and places where two mobility days in a week makes sense. Just depends on how much you're crushing it.

Gerald Poole:

Yeah. And there are many unique things that you'll put into either a regular workout or a mobility day that are ... I'll use the term "***underrated***," even though I'm not certain they are. Because I don't know too much about who else uses them.

Stewart Smith:

Absolutely, I agree with everything you're doing. Your WHYS, I think, are not only just fun challenges to get you to these events, and accomplish some things that you want to accomplish. But in the end, they're going to help you with your ability to be the guy who can help people. I want you to know, this is what I think it should come down to for all of us – to be able to help people. As well as help yourself, too. Because there are those times, too, you have to be able to help yourself, in certain situations.

And the one thing, too, is don't forget that fitness is a journey, and not a destination. There's no, "***Okay, I'm done. I've reached my _____*** " Like you said, it is a hobby. It should be considered a hobby. Experiment with different programs. Learn how to train. Learn how to cycle through different elements of fitness. And we're talking about all the elements of fitness. We're talking about endurance. Strength. Muscle stamina. Flexibility. Mobility. Speed and agility. **Periodization Training** - All of those things are elements that we need to be better tactical athletes. And we have to be good at all of them. There can't be one that we cannot do, and be considered a ready tactical athlete.

For instance, if you can't swim, you are ineffective on 75% of this earth, which is a horrible thing to think about. And there are many people who cannot swim. Take a lesson at a local YMCA. Take a beginner kids' lesson if you need to, if you're an adult. There's nothing wrong with just getting an instructor, and learning how to swim.

Gerald Poole: Stew, I just want to say, real quickly, it helps to know that people like you (Navy SEALs) struggle with things too. You think certain people don't have flaws or weaknesses and are good at everything, and I started learning that, no, everybody has things they need to work on. Everybody has things they want to get improve upon. Everybody has things they've failed. And as soon as you start realizing that, it helps make it more doable.

It's something that we all face. You're not unique in that you failed. You're not unique in that you need to lose 20 pounds and get off the couch, and you haven't run. Or whatever it is. You just have to start doing it.

And the kindness piece, too. I think kindness is so underrated. And when you talk about helping people, I think that's another source of happiness also.

Stewart Smith: Well, I will say this. I think we've hit all the things I wanted to hit in this conversation. Now, the rest of this project is—as you read on—will be exercises, workouts, arranged in a way where I'm going to phase this thing out. And this one's for beginners. And we're going to rebuild you, if you are injured, and we're going to focus on all the different elements of fitness. And it may take some time, but be patient, because I will promise you, in a year from now - think about this. Think about where you were last year, at this time. Last Thanksgiving, or wherever we were. And it's just like yesterday. So, a year from now, you will wish you had started today.

Gerald Poole: Absolutely. And like you said, it's a journey. It's a succession of successful workouts. A succession of successful days. A succession of successful weeks and months. It's not going to happen tomorrow, but accept that, and have fun with it. And that's really what's brought me happiness. I may not even be halfway there. I'm excited to know that I'm going to go back and crush these goals, and that I'm going to be so much more fit a year from now, and two years from now, than where I am today. And yeah, I'm anxious to meet my goals, but it might take another two years. It might take ... I don't know how long. I don't care. It's the process that I've really started to focus on, and fall in love with.

Stewart Smith: There you go. I love that. Because, do what you like to do first. Whatever gets you into the weight room. Whatever gets you into the gym. Whatever exercise. You like to bench-press? Make sure there's bench-press every day when you go into the workout ... Well, not every day, but every other day, you should be doing bench-press as part of your workout. You love to bench-press? Do it.

But then start adding some supplemental training that help balance out what you like and what gets you into the weight room. Also work your lower body. Work your upper back. Work your core. Work your cardio. All of those things. Otherwise it makes this journey a little more difficult. But there are also many things that I didn't like before, because I'd never tried them. You have to go try it. See if you like it.

Stewart Smith: Give it a shot. Next thing you know, you're going to be on this new journey. And it might be triathlons. It might be marathons. It might be GORUCK challenges. It might be the SEALFIT challenge. It might be one of our Special Ops Triathlons. Whatever those goals are that you have can grow from every day just getting into the weight room, building some persistence. And having a little bit of motivation at first, but eventually, that motivation is going to evolve into habits that you've created. And when you can't rely on your motivation, what do you rely on?

Gerald Poole: Your discipline.

Stewart Smith: Discipline. You have disciplined yourself through all these persistent daily challenges that you've gone through that now you say, "***Well, I'm not really*** *motivated to work out, but I'm going to go work out anyway."*

Gerald Poole: Which happens a lot.

Stewart Smith: Absolutely. There are many times I don't feel like getting up at 5:15 and working out with guys 20 years younger than me. But, I know I always will feel better after doing it. And that's the key. So, Gerald, I want to thank you so much for your time. For doing this for me. Because, like I said, your story is so common. So common, about people who've had a different background, but now have similar goals of being there for people. And being able to provide assistance if needed. Or be able to just plain help yourself.

Stewart Smith: One day, I want you to say, and to anybody who's reading this or listening to this, is to say that, "My fitness level saved my life." And don't let it be the reason why you die, or the reason why you were unable to help someone you love. That's how important fitness is. And that's what tactical fitness is.

Gerald Poole: Absolutely, man. And that's part of it for me, too.

Stewart Smith: Yeah. I love it. So, hey, Gerald, thank you so much.

Stewart Smith: ## **<u>Now let's get to work!</u>**

Getting Started

The following stretching plan will assist you with getting started again safely and without as much post-exercise soreness.

Most injuries are strains or muscle pulls that can be prevented with a few simple stretching exercises done daily. The added flexibility will not only assist in injury prevention, but with speed workouts and help you to run faster. The following is a stretching routine that can be used whether you are a beginner or advanced athlete.

The Warm-Up Routine

Finding what works best for you as a warm-up is critical to your success in either fitness testing as well as long term job performance. Increasing your flexibility should be the first goal before starting fitness/athletic activity. This dynamic stretch routine is a quick and effective way to warm up prior to your workout as well as cooldown in the pool afterwards to produce the desired results of mobility and flexibility.

Chapter Four: Dynamic Stretching and Core Exercises

A quick and easy to follow dynamic stretching routine will demonstrate the way to warm up and prepare for workouts. Take 5-10 minutes and get warmed up with these leg movements prior to working out. You can do this one on land (typically) or add a session in chest deep water. Click the hyper link to see most of these in motion.

> **Jog or Bike - 5 minutes**
> **Butt Kickers - 1 minute**
> **Frankenstein Walks - 1 minute**
> **Bounding in Place - 1 minute**
> **Side Steps with hip opener – 1 min**
> **Leg Swings Front / Back– 1 minute**
> **Leg Swings (Left / Right) – 1 minute**
> **Calf/Shin Warm-up – 1 minute**
> **Burpees – 1 minute**
> **Light Arm Shoulder Chest Stretch**
> **Light Thigh Stretch**
> **Light Hamstring Stretch**
> **Back Roll**
> **Light ITB Roll**
> **Shin Roll**

Warming Up / Cooling Down for Workouts

Jog five minutes or do a series of light calisthenics like jumping jacks, crunches, push-ups, or squats prior to stretching. Dynamic stretching is a major part of warming up prior to any athletic movements. In order to reduce muscle fatigue and soreness and perhaps prevent injuries, perform a good warm-up using these dynamic/static stretches. You can also use these on the back end of a hard workout to cool-down from hard activity. Perform in the pool for even better results as a cool down. ***However, you can do this on land if you do not have a pool.***

Jog or Bike 5 minutes – Get the blood flowing.

<u>Butt Kickers</u> - **1 minute:** Jog slowly and flex your hamstrings to pull your heels to your butt on each step. Do with knees down then with knees up for 30-60 seconds.

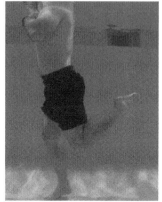

<u>Frankenstein Walks</u> - **1 minute:** Walk and kick high each step. Try to kick your hands in front of you. Do 10 kicks with each leg.

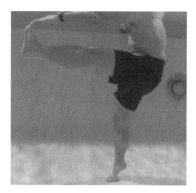

Bounding - 1 minute: Do high powered skipping for 1 minute. Start off with regular skipping then lift knees high each step. Do in place for 1 minute

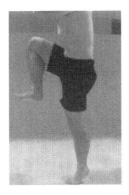

Side steps w / hips openers - 30 seconds each direction: Work lateral movement into the warm-up. Step sideways by lifting the leg and opening the hip to the side you step. Do for 1 minute back and forth alternating in each direction.

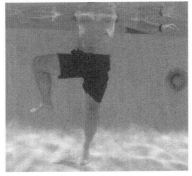

Leg swings – 1 minute: Stand still and lift legs back and forth with legs straight at full range of motion of your hip (front / back). Then swing leg left and right in front of your body for 10 reps each leg.

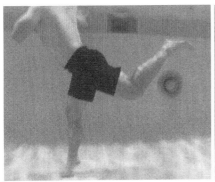
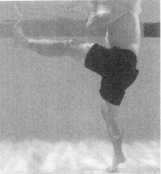

Side Leg swings – 1 minute: Stand still and lift legs back and forth with legs straight at full range of motion of your hip side to side (left / right).

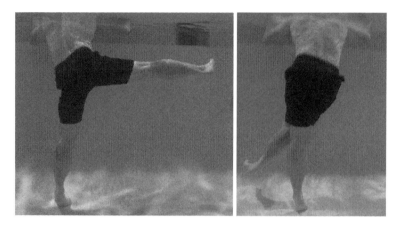

Calf/Shin Warm-up – 1 minute: Alternate lifting heels off the floor and toes off the floor. This is a shins/calves builder to help strengthen legs for running/rucking.

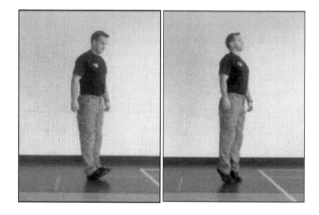

Burpees – 1 minute: Drop into the pushup position. Quickly drop your chest to the floor and back to the up position. Bring your feet up and stand and jump 4-6" off the ground to finish the rep.

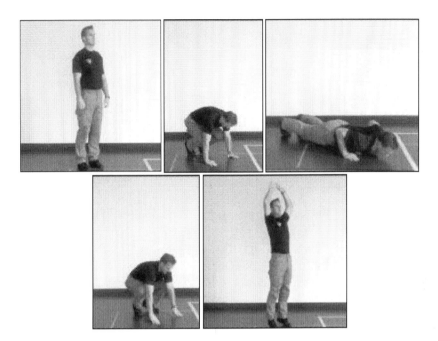

Light Arm Shoulder/Chest stretch: Pull your arm across your torso to stretch rear/deltoid and trapezius region. Then pull your arms backward as far as you can to stretch the chest/front shoulder connections.

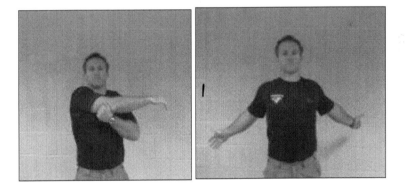

Thigh Stretch – Standing: - Standing, bend your knee and grab your foot at the ankle. Pull your heel to your butt and push your hips forward. Hold for 10-15 seconds and repeat with the other leg.

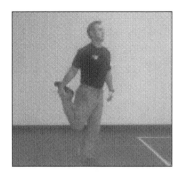

Hamstring Stretch #1: - From the standing position, bend forward at the waist and come close to touching your toes, slightly bend your knees. Go back and forth from straight legs to bent knees to feel the top/bottom part of the hamstring stretch. You should feel this stretching the back of your thighs.

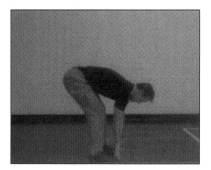

More Stretching Plans

There is a supplemental stretching plan full of exercises that can be found in the lower back plan (legs, hips, core). In an effort to save space, for pictures of static stretches, check out the PDF file:

Lower Back Plan

http://site.stewsmithptclub.com/lowerbackplan.pdf

Foam Rolling - <u>Myofascial Release</u> <u>Foam Roller Article / Video</u>

<u>Back roll</u>: Sit on foam roller and move slowly back and forth as you lie on the roller. Move your legs to move your body over the roller. Do for 1-2 minutes each body part.

<u>ITB roll:</u> Lay on your side in a side plank position and place foam roller under your hip. Move forward and roll your ITB from the hip to below the knee. Do for 1-2 minutes on each side of the leg.

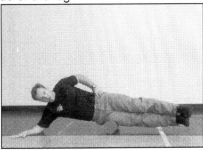

<u>Shin Roll:</u> Place roller under your knees and slowly kneel down placing both shins on the roller. Slowly roll back and forth from bottom on the knee to the top of the ankle.

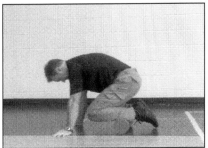

<u>More Foam Rolling Ideas</u>

Core Workout Exercises

Abdominal exercises as a warm up before/after stretching

When you exercise your stomach muscles, make sure to exercise and stretch your back also. The stomach and lower back muscles are opposing muscle groups and if one is much stronger than the other, you can injure the weaker muscle group easily.

The Crunch (Core) Cycle – When you see the term CRUNCH CYCLE, it means you will do a series of these core exercises. We recommend doing all the core exercises in this section for 10-20 repetitions – just one time through. If you cannot do all of the repetitions or exercises, just skip, one day you will. See chart below:

Crunch (Core) Cycle:
Crunches 10-20
Reverse Crunches 10-20
Double Crunches 10-20
Left Crunches 10-20
Right Crunches 10-20
Bicycle Crunches 10-20
Swimmers 30-60 seconds
Hip Rollers 10 each side
Arm hauler 20
Reverse Pushups 20
Birds 20
Plank pose 1 min

Advanced Crunch - (Legs up): Lie on your back with your feet straight in the air. Keep your legs straight up in the air for the advanced crunches. Cross your hands over your chest and bring your elbows to your knees by flexing your stomach.

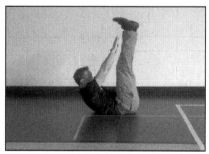

Reverse Crunch: In the same position as the regular crunch, lift your knees and butt toward your elbows. Leave your head and upper body flat on the ground. Only move your legs and butt.

(Do not do if you have severe lower back injury or if this hurts your back)

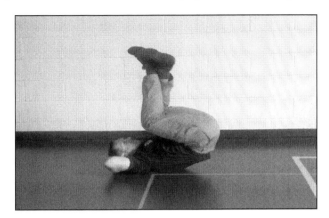

Double Crunch: Lift hips and shoulders off the floor at the same time in one motion.

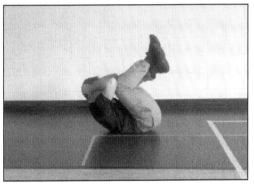

Right Elbow to Left Knee: Cross your left leg over your right leg. Flex your stomach and twist to bring your right elbow to your left knee.

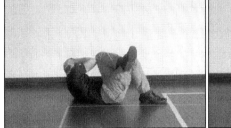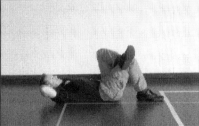

Left Elbow to Right Knee: Cross your right leg over your leg. Flex your stomach and twist to bring your left elbow to your right knee.

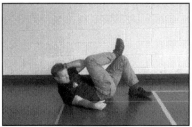 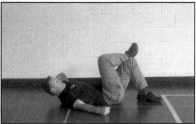

Bicycles: This is a mix between opposite elbow to knee crunches with bicycling of your legs. Alternate from side to side for prescribed reps and do not let feet touch the floor.

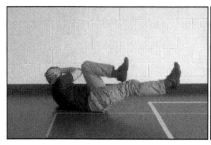 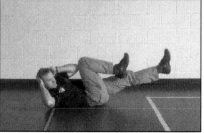

Lower Back Exercise - Swimmers: Lie on your stomach and lift your feet and knees off the floor by flutter kicking repeatedly as if you were swimming freestyle – build up to 1:00 – or keep feet still but off the floor.

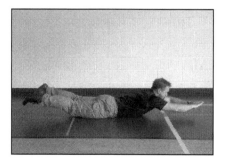

Lower Back Exercise #2 - Hip Rolls: Lie flat on your back with your knees in the air as in the middle picture below. Keep your shoulders on the floor, rotate your hips and legs to the left and right as shown below.

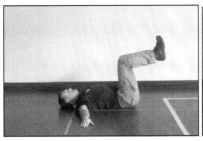 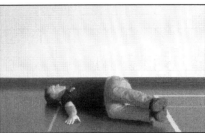

Upper back exercise #1 - Arm Haulers: Lie on your stomach. Lift your chest slightly off the floor and wave your arms from your sides to over your head for 30 seconds.

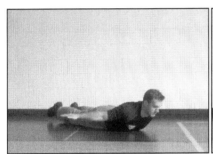 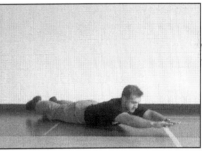

Upper back exercise #2 - Reverse Push-ups - Lie on your stomach in the down push-up position. Lift your hands off the floor instead of pushing the floor. This will strengthen your upper back muscles that oppose the chest muscles.

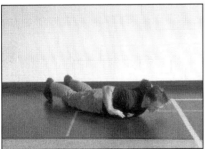 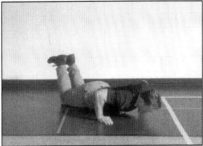

Upper back exercise #3 – Birds: Lie on your stomach with your arms spread to the height of your shoulders. Lift both arms off the floor until your shoulder blades "pinch" and place them slowly in the down position. Repeat for 10-15 repetitions mimicking a bird flying.

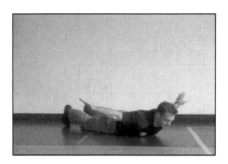

Plank Pose and One Arm Plank: To complete the Crunch Cycle, try getting into the plank position and see if you can hold it for at least 1 minute. As you advance, lean on the left / right arm as you increase the time. Or do the plank in the UP Pushup position.

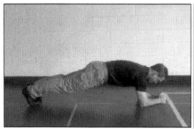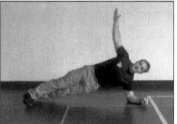

In fact, when you fail at pushups during the workout, stay in the UP Pushup position for an extra 30-60 seconds each time. This will prepare you well for the long periods of time in the "leaning rest" as well as strengthen the core for crawling obstacles.

Chapter Five: Upper Body Calisthenics Exercises

<u>Regular Push-ups</u> - Lie on the ground with your hands placed flat next to your chest. Your hands should be about shoulder width apart. Push yourself up by straightening your arms and keeping your back stiff. Look forward as you perform this exercise. *(You can also mix in wide and close stance pushups for variety if you prefer.)*

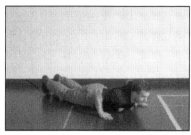 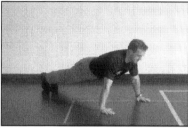

<u>Parallel Bar dips</u> - Grab the bars with your hands and put all of your weight on your arms and shoulders. Do not do these exercises with added weight, if you are a beginner, or if you have had a previous shoulder injury. **To complete the exercise, bring yourself down so your elbows form a 90 degree angle (no less of an angle) and back to the up position.**

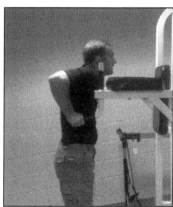 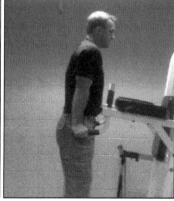

Get good at pull-ups and dips as they will help you pull yourself up and over climbing obstacles when faced with a wall, rope, or ladder climb.

Pull-ups (regular grip) - Grab the pull-up bar with your hands placed about shoulder width apart and your palms facing away from you. Pull yourself upward until your chin is over the bar and complete the exercise by slowly moving to the hanging position.

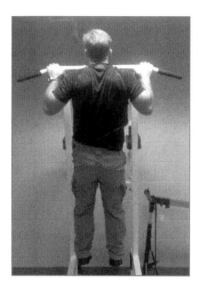

Mix in different grips for a variety (wide grip, close grip, alternated grip) *Note – When using a reverse grip - keep your hands in and do not go wider than your shoulders as you will develop some elbow tendonitis similar to that of tennis elbow.

When you fail at pullups, add in DB rows, assisted pullups, or pulldowns to complete the set

Squats - Keep your feet shoulder width apart. Drop your butt back as though sitting in a chair. Concentrate on squeezing your glutes in your upward motion. Keep your heels on the ground and knees over your ankles. Your shins should be near vertical at all times. Extend your buttocks backward. Do with or without a dumbbell / kettlebell in your hands.

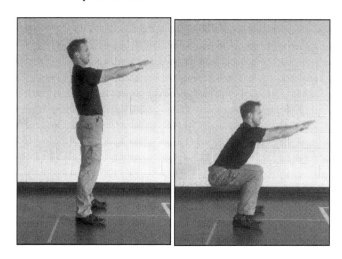

Walking Lunge - Keep your chest up high and your stomach tight. Take a long step forward and drop your back knee toward the ground. Stand up on your forward leg, bringing your feet together and repeat with the other leg. Make sure your knee never extends past your foot. Keep your shin vertical in other words.

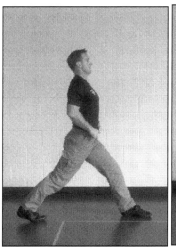
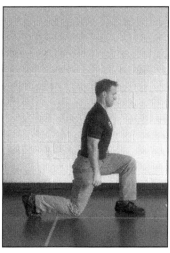

Chapter Six: Dumbbell and Weighted Exercises

Bench Press: Lie on your back on a bench, placing the legs bent with feet flat on the floor on both sides of the bench. Extend your arms upward, grab the machine, barbell, or dumbbells just greater than shoulder width and lower the bar to your chest slowly. The bar should hit just below the nipples on your sternum. Extend your arms again to a locked position and repeat several times.

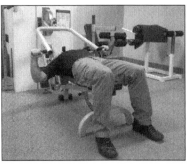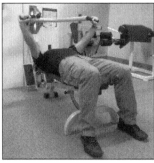

Pull-down Machine – This is an easier form of pull-ups, but you have to start somewhere. Using a pull-down machine, grab the bar, sit down and pull the bar to your collar bones. Keep the bar in front of you. Keep the bar moving in front of your body / not behind your head. **Change grips as you can on the pull-up bar (wide, regular, close and reverse).**

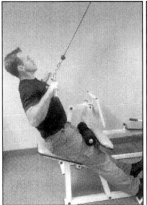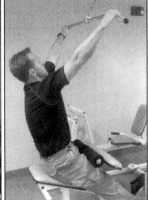

DB rows – Grab dumbbell (DB) in one hand and lean forward onto a bench supporting your back with your opposite knee and hand on the bench. Pull the DB up to your chest, hold for 1 second and slowly extend arm. Repeat 10/arm.

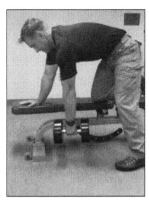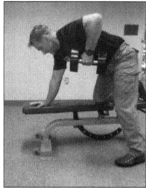

Wood Chopper Squat with Dumbbell – Add a dumbbell to the squat by swinging the weight over your head when standing and between your legs when squatting. Keep head up and back straight.

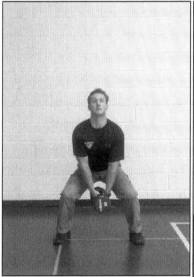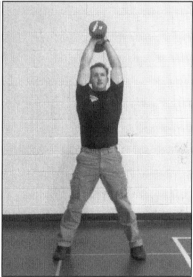

Kettle bell swing – Similar to the woodchopper squat, except for less squat and more hip and torso movement, explode with your legs and hips to get the kettlebell or dumbbell above your head.

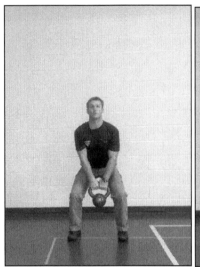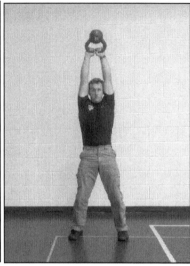

MJDB #1 - Multi-Joint Dumbbell Exercise: Perform a bicep curl, then press the dumbbells over your head with a military press, and then go straight into a triceps extension - repeat in reverse order to get to the starting position.

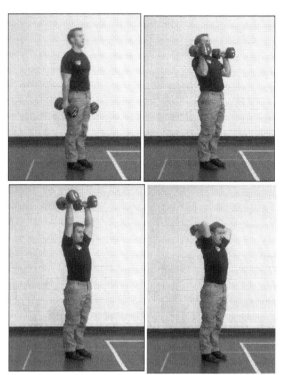

MJDB #2: Same as above but add in a squat when your hands are in the down bicep position (by your hips)

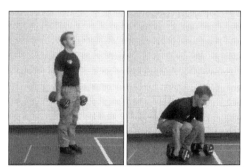

Same as MJDB#1 plus a squat / deadlift

Thruster (front squat into over head press) – Explode upward from the front squat position straight into an overhead press or push press.

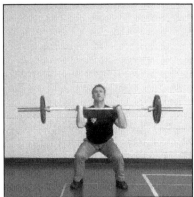 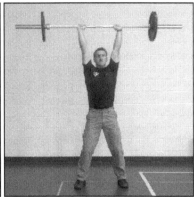

* The thruster is a deeper version of the "Push Press" exercise. You can opt to do the Push Press if you burn out with doing full squats but still have upper body left in the set.

Thrusters with dumbbells – You can do these with dumbbells as well or even a single plate. The goal is to squat and forcefully stand and use the momentum of the upward movement to easily lift the weight over your head

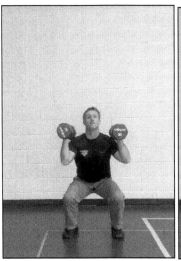 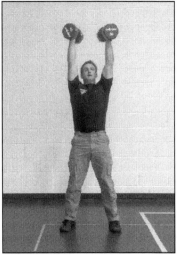

Farmer Walk – Grab a weight or sandbag with a handle in one hand and walk 100m changing hands at the 50m mark. This is great for grip as well as core strength.

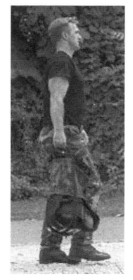

Chapter Seven: The Light Weight Shoulder Workout

This shoulder routine is great for post rotator cuff / shoulder surgery physical therapy patients. <u>See link to video</u> that explains all of the exercises in actual progression.

LATERAL RAISE: More than 5 pound dumbbells is not recommended for this exercise. Keep your shoulders back and your chest high. Lift weights parallel to ground in a smooth controlled motion, keep your palms facing the ground. Follow the next 6 exercises without stopping.

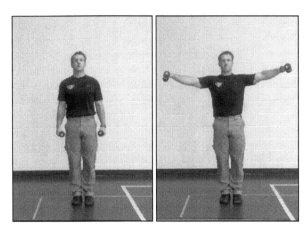

THUMBS UP: After performing 10 regular lateral raises, do 10 lateral raises with your thumbs up, touching your hips with your palms facing away from you and raising your arms no higher than shoulder height.

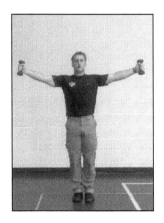

THUMBS-UP/DOWN: Continue with side lateral raises. As you lift your arms upward, keep your thumbs up. Once your arms are shoulder height, turn your hands and make your thumbs point toward the floor. Repeat for 10 times, always leading in the up and down direction with your thumbs.

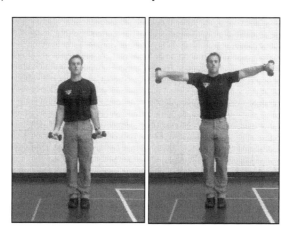

FRONT RAISE - THUMBS-UP: Now, for 10 more repetitions, to work your front deltoids. Lift the dumbbells from your waist to shoulder height keeping your thumbs up and arms straight.

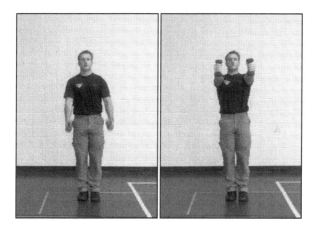

CROSS-OVERS: With your palms facing away from you and arms relaxed in front of your hips, bring your arms up and over your head as if you were doing a jumping jack (without jumping). Cross your arms IN FRONT of your head and bring them back to your hips for 10 repetitions.

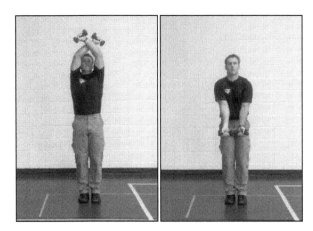

MILITARY PRESS: Place one foot ahead of the other as shown and knees slightly bent to reduce strain on your lower back. Exhale as you push the weights over your head for 10 final repetitions in the mega-shoulder pump workout. Slowly lower them to shoulder height and repeat. Muscles used are shoulders and triceps (back of arm).

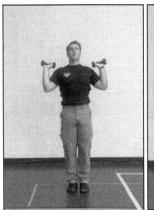
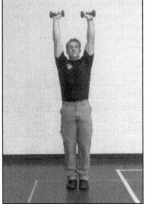

Section Three: Workouts and Explanations

This section is to help explain some of the workout designs. The goal in these workouts is to do what you can or have time for. If you do not have a pool, try another form of non-impact cardio options. If you have a pool but do not swim, try swimming some, but focus on the treading and dynamic stretching in the pool as this is exceptional for your hips, legs, and lower back. You can also work your shoulders and elbows as well by doing jumping jacks or other underwater movements with your arms to work your joints in a full range of motion.

Warmup / Stretch
You will see a Warmup 5-10 minutes / stretch at the start of your workouts. This can be whatever you prefer. You can do it with a bike, jog, walk or other quick cardio event or the squat or pushup pyramid / short run warmup.

PT Pyramid Warmups – Find a place to do 15-25m run or dynamic stretches in between exercises. Often burpee pyramid, squat / pushup pyramids will make up the warmup pyramid. Do 1 rep of exercise – run 25meters – do 2 reps, run 25m..usually the pyramid will only go up to 5 or 10 sets. A good place to do the short runs is a basketball court, tennis court, or field. You do not have to repeat in reverse order down the pyramid unless it states. Mix in some dynamic stretches during the 25m sections (buttkickers, frankensteins, side steps, high knees, side steps, etc.. Once you get to 10 – you are done with the warmup. Usually the set will be from 5-10 and depicted as such: ***Run / Pushup Pyramid 1-10.***

Circuit Workouts - You will see several different circuit routines in this workout program. Basically, a circuit workout is designed to move you as quickly through a workout as possible. There are no rest periods in a circuit until the end. Moving from one exercise to the other is the only rest you will get, but you will rarely be using the same muscle group two times in a row. There is actually rest built into the workout. If you have to rearrange the circuit order, that is fine to fit into your weight room if busy.

PT with the clock - This type of workout is designed to help students ace a physical fitness test of pullups, pushups, and sit-ups. By performing as many reps as you can of each exercise in a certain time limit, you will be learning the pace required to achieve as many pushups and sit-ups in 1-2 minutes possible. By using the clock as your training guide, you will become accustomed to doing maximum reps in a time period which will further increase your scores as you continue to practice this type of training.

Tabata Intervals – Do 20 second sprint / 10 second easy for timed sets in the workout – usually done on bike, elliptical, or rowing machines.

Life Cycle Workout – Riding a stationary bike with increasing resistance levels, place bike on manual mode. Start off at level 1 or 2 and increase the resistance every minute until failure. Then repeat in reverse order. If your bike increases up to 20 levels – increase resistance by 2 levels every minute. Otherwise, just increase by one level if bike tops out at 10-12 levels.

Extra Weekend Cardio – Over the course of Friday, Saturday, and Sunday, try to accumulate _____ minutes (will progress each week) over the weekend. The time can be completed with 10 minute walks after each meal or long walks of the dog, etc.

If you have a pool...Consider Treading Water <u>(video options)</u>

Pool Mobility Day Off <u>(full article)</u>

Tread water for 10 minutes – Work on big scissor kicks, breast stroke kicks, and arm range of motion strokes (like jumping jacks off the bottom of the pool).

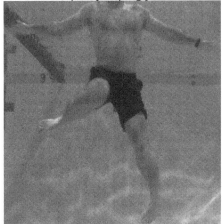

Then, like you do before you run with a warmup with a variety of dynamic stretches:

Try all dynamic stretches you do but in the pool in about chest-deep water (butt-kickers, Frankenstein walks, high knee lifts, leg swings (front / back / side to side).

Swim or tread water - 5 minutes

Butt Kickers - 1 minute

Frankenstein Walks - 1 minute

High Knee / Hip openers - 1 minute

Side Steps with hip opener – 1 min

Leg Swings Front / Back– 1 minute

Leg Swings (Left / Right) – 1 minute

(repeat with more options or longer time if needed)

Sequence of events for Swim Mobility Drills
Swim 5:00
Treading – 5:00
Dynamic stretches 5:00 in chest deep water.

If you do not have a pool, you can repeat the dynamic stretches and static stretches on land if you prefer to cool down with some mobility work.

The Program

This Tactical Fitness program will challenge you and may push you to failure many days. But, there are recovery days built into the middle of the week on Day 3 or Day 4. You still want workouts that will push your perceived limits, but you need at least one day off per week (5-6 workouts / week) and one of those days can be a Recovery Day. This is challenging, but not impossible. I promise you that you will be amazed at what you can do after you complete this twelve week course. Do the stretches, foam rolling, dynamic warmups and water time for best results.

Running Replacement

During the beginning phases of ANY workout, some people need LESS running mileage when starting a workout plan. If you are finding the running / speed workouts to be too much replace some of the runs with equal timed non-impact cardio events such as bike pyramid, elliptical and rowing tabata intervals, and swimming using the Running Non-Impact Replacement.

Good luck with the program and remember to consult your physician first before starting any program if you have not exercised in several months or years. If you need help with any fitness related questions please feel free to email me at stew@stewsmith.com.

The Workouts

The charts below contain twelve weeks of workouts to help you rebuild that fitness foundation and better prepare for the life after 40. The goal on starting after a long period of time without training or if this is your first-time training, is to TREAT YOURSELF LIKE A BEGINNER. This is what Phase 1 is all about. Give it 21 days to build a new habit of easy fitness without getting too sore, injured, or burned out. Building a foundation of fitness is all about building a new habit of moving. Eventually this motivation to train will become a habit and your own discipline will drive the growth of your abilities.

ABOUT the 21 Day Habit Building Program:

Beginner Cycle: Days 1-21: Calisthenics / Weight Training Mix and Non impact cardio.

- The goal here is the do some form of activity daily for these first 21 days – even if that is just walking for 10 minutes after every meal.

Weeks 4-6: Calisthenics and Weights Mix Foundation Building With Cardio (Running Optional)

Weeks 7-12: Transition into Calisthenics / DBs Only and Running and / or Non-Impact Cardio Progression

Enjoy the workout charts below. They will challenge you and help you perform like you did decades before:

The 21-Day Habit Foundation Building Program

Day 1	Day 2	Day 3
Day 1 **Crunch Cycle -10 each** **Squats 25 total** while walking up/down stairs *Walk or bike 15:00	**Day 2** **Repeat 5x's** Pushups -10 / MJDB#1-10 Squats - 10 **Shoulder workout** **Walk or bike 15:00**	**Day 3** Crunch Cycle Circuit -10 **Mini-Mobility Day** **Repeat 3 times** Bike, row, elliptical 5 min Roam roll or stretch 5 min
Day 4 **Repeat 5 times** Pushups 5-10 Bicep curl/tricep ext–10 **Shoulder workout** Walk / run/bike - 15:00	**Day 5** **Crunch Cycle 10 each** Walk / run/bike - 15:00	**Day 6 Repeat 5x's** Walk / run/ bike - 4:00 squats - 20 / lunges - 10
Day 7 Crunch Cycle Circuit -10 **Mini-Mobility Day** **Repeat 3 times** Bike, row, elliptical 5 min Roam roll or stretch 5 min	**Day 8** **Repeat 5 times** Jumping jacks - 10 Pushups - 10 (no rest) Shoulder Workout	**Day 9** **Repeat 3 times** Walk or bike 5:00 squats - 20 lunge-10/leg
Day 10 **Crunch Cycle 15 reps** **Shoulder workout** walk / run / bike - 15:00	**Day 11 Repeat 3 times** Plank pose – 1:00 Bench dips – 5-10 Walk or bike - 15:00	**Day 12 Repeat 5x's** Jumping jacks - 10 Pushups – 10 **Shoulder workout**
Day 13 **Crunch Cycle -15 reps** Squats – 3 x 15 reps Walk or bike - 15:00	**Day 14** **Repeat 4x's** jumping jacks - 10 Pushups – 10 **Shoulder Workout**	**Day 15** Crunch Cycle Circuit -10 **Mini-Mobility Day** **Repeat 3 times** Bike, row, elliptical 5 min Roam roll or stretch 5 min
Day 16 **Repeat 5x's** MJDB#2 - 10 squats - 10 / lunges 10 **Shoulder Workout**	**Day 17** **Crunch Cycle 15 reps** Walk or bike - 15:00	**Day 18** **Repeat 4x's** Pushups - 10 Squats –15 **Shoulder Workout**
Day 19 **Crunch Cycle 15 reps** walk / run / bike - 15:00	**Day 20** **Repeat 5x's** Pushups - 10 Squats - 20/crunch- 20	**Day 21** **Crunch cycle 15 reps** **Squat 50 total** during walk or bike 20:00

*Every day – Stretch 10 minutes after exercise – head to toe

Spring - Week 4 – Calisthenics / Weights Mix – Running Optional		
Day 1	Day 2	Day 3
Upper body Workout Warm-up bike / walk - total 10:00 / Stretch **Repeat 5 times** jumping jacks 10 crunches 10 pushups 10 Light weight Shoulder **Repeat 3-4x's** Cardio - 5:00 - but make each minute harder than the previous (increase speed, resistance) MJDB#1 – 10 reps crunches - 25 pushups - 10-15 plank pose 1 min DB Rows - 15 reps Light weight Shoulder Walk/jog mix or bike, elliptical, rower, swim 15-20 minute cool-down Stretch	Lowerback plan – Core and Stretches Long Cardio / Legs Your choice - 45-60 minutes of any mix of bike, walk/run, or other cardio mixes - but every 10 minutes - stop and do 20 squats / 10 lunges	Walk or jog 5:00 light stretch Light weight Shoulder **Repeat 3 times** walk/jog or bike 5 min Bench press 10 military press 10 MJDB#1 - 10-15 rep DB rows 10-15 pushups 10-15 crunches 25 plank pose 1 minute Light weight Shoulder Walk/jog mix 15-20 minute cool-down Stretch

Week 4 - Calisthenics Weights Mix – Running Optional		
Day 4	Day 5	Day 6
Mobility Day **Repeat 5 times** Any non impact cardio (bike, elliptical, row, swim) 5 minutes Foam roll or stretch 5 minutes **If pool available:** swim 5 minutes tread 5 minutes dynamic stretches in water 5 minutes If no pool do stretches in the Lower Back Plan	Full body LWS - 5 lbs **Repeat 5 times** jumping jacks 10 squats 10 crunches 10 pushups 10 Pull / Leg Workout: **Repeat 3 times** pullups max OR DB rows 10/arm DB bicep curls 10/arm Leg press 10 or DB squats 10 **Repeat 5 times** jumping jacks 10 pushups 5-10 crunches 20 Push / Leg Workout **Repeat 3 times** Pushups 10-15 reps DB chest press 10 lunges 10/leg bench dips 10 MJDB#1 - 10 Lightweight shoulder Cardio Cooldown - 30 minutes of steady cardio - walk, bike, jog, etc...	Weekend walks – How much can you walk this weekend? Walk in the AM____ 10 min walks after meals _____ Walk in the PM____ Can you get 1-2 hours worth of walking or other cardio options? And stretch 10 minutes each day over the weekend

Week 5 - Calisthenics / Weights Mix – Running Optional		
Day 1	Day 2	Day 3
Warmup with 1-10 Pushup pyramid - walk/jog 25yards do 1 pushup, walk.jog 25yds do 2 pushups...up to 10 / stretch. Lightweight shoulders **Repeat 3x's** MJDB#2 - 10reps crunches -25 pushups - 10-15 plank pose 1 min Squats 10 DB Rows - 10/arm **PT Reset:** Reverse Pushups 10 Birds 10 Arm Haulers 10 Walk 15-20 minute cool-down	Lowerback Plan **Long Cardio** Your choice - 45-60 minutes of any mix of bike, walk/run.	Mobility Day **Repeat 5 times** Any non impact cardio (bike, elliptical, row, swim) 5 minutes Foam roll or stretch 5 minutes **If pool available:** swim 5 minutes tread 5 minutes dynamic stretches in water 5 minutes If no pool do stretches in the Lower Back Plan

Week 5 - Calisthenics / Weights Mix – Running Optional		
Day 4	Day 5	Day 6
Squat / pushups pyramid: squat 1 / pushups 1 run 25m. squat 2 / pushups 2 run 25m...keep going up until you fail at pushups - stop at 10. *do on basketball court, field, driveway etc.. **Repeat 3 times** Pushups max DB rows 10/arm Lunges 10/leg MJDB#2 - 10reps Situps or crunches 20 **PT Reset:** Reverse Pushups 10 Birds 10 Arm Haulers 10 Walk 15-20 minute cool-down	Lowerback Plan Long Cardio Take a long walk or walk/run combo today - or bike for as long as you have time. 30min? 45min? 1 hour? plus?	Warmup with 5-10 min easy walk/jog Lightweight shoulders **Repeat 5 times** Jumping jacks 10 Pushups 5 Plank pose 15 secs Squats 10 **Repeat 3 times** Military press 10 DB rows 10 Step up 5 / leg MJDB#2 - 10 Crunches 20 3 min fast / slow interval walk/jog OR NOT....just slow if needed. Cardio Cooldown - 15 minutes of steady cardio - walk, bike, jog, etc...

Week 6 - Calisthenics / Weights Mix – Running Optional		
Day 1	Day 2	Day 3
Push, Pull, Core, Cardio Pushups Pyramid 1-5 - run 25m in between: 1 pushup - walk/run 25m, 2 pushups...stop at 5. **1 min sets TEST:** Pushups 1 min Pullups 1max - any? Situps 1 min or plank pose 1 min Cardio 5 min - How far do you get in 5 min of any cardio? **Repeat 3 times** Bench press 10 Pulldowns 10 Reverse Pushups 10 Birds 10 Arm Haulers 10 Cardio 5 min Lightweight Shoulder Walk, jog, swim, or bike 20 minutes for max distance.	Leg Day Squat pyramid 1-10 - run /walk 25m in btwn: 1 squat - 25m, 2 squats - 25m...stop at 10. For intermediate level: Squat pyramid 1-10 up/down flight of stairs: 1 squat - run up/down stairs, 2 squats up/down stairs...up to 10 - stop. **Repeat 3 times** Bike, walk, or row 3 min fast Leg ext 10 Leg curl 10 or squats 20 (air) Leg press 10 (if available) How far can you bike, elliptical, or row for 15 minutes?	Cardio Day Pick one for 30 minutes of pick and choose combinations for 30-40 minutes total: Bike or walk, or walk/jog mix 15 minute warmup **15min of fast / slow:** 1 min fast / 1 min slow of the above choice of warm up. Or walk 10 minutes after every meal in your day if too busy

Week 6 - Calisthenics / Weights Mix – Running Optional		
Day 4	Day 5	Day 6
Full Body **Warmup with 5 min cardio options / light stretch** **Repeat 3 times** Jumping jacks 10 pushups 5-10 Crunches 10-20 Squats 10 **Lightweight Shoulder** **Repeat 3 times** Cardio 5 min Pushups 10 DB rows 10 Farmer walk up/down stairs 3x MJDB#2 - 10 Plank pose 1 min Cardio 15-20 min of walk, jog, bike, mix in a pyramid (every minute gets tougher with increase of resistance, incline or speed - start easy - end easy)	Mobility Day **Repeat 5 times** Any non impact cardio (bike, elliptical, row, swim) 5 minutes Foam roll or stretch 5 minutes **If pool available:** swim 5 minutes tread 5 minutes dynamic stretches in water 5 minutes If no pool do stretches in the Lower Back Plan	Cardio Weekend Try to mix in 60-90 minutes spread through the weekend of some sort of movement: walk, jog, bike, elliptical, swim, or other form of movement. Even if you break it up with 10 minute walks after meals or long walks of the dog. Get out and move.

Week 7-12: Calisthenics and Weights Progression / Cardio Options

Week 7 - Calisthenics / Weights Progression – Cardio		
Day 1	Day 2	Day 3
Pushup / Squat pyramid 1-5 warmup - run 25m 1 pushup / 1 squat, run 25m 2 pushups, 2 squats...keep going to 5/5. **Repeat 5 times** Jumping jacks 10 Pushups 5-10 Squats 10 **Repeat 3 times** Pullups max OR DB rows 10/arm Pushups or Db bench 5-10 Squats 10-20 (air) Lunges 10/leg crunches 25 plank pose 1 min Cooldown cardio 15-20 minutes of walk, bike, jog..etc, Your choice for max distance.	Cardio 20 min bike Pyramid - each minute is tougher than previous minute. IF AVAILABLE 20 min walk/run combo or walk longer if you prefer. **Upper Core Spread throughout day:** **Repeat 2 times** Reverse pushups 10 Birds 10 Arm Haulers 10 - Plank Pose 1 min Lower back plan - do it later in the evening	Pushup / Squat pyramid 1-5 warmup - run 25m 1 pushup / 1 squat, run 25m 2 pushups, 2 squats...keep going to 5/5. **Repeat 3 times** Pushups 10-15 DB bench 10 Pullups - max? or DB rows 10/arm MJDB#2 - 10 Lighter Weight **Repeat 3 times** DB Military press 10 DB Squats 10 Light weight shoulders Cooldown cardio 15-20 minutes of walk, bike, jog..etc, Your choice for max distance.

Week 7 - Calisthenics / Weights Progression – Cardio		
Day 4	Day 5	Day 6
Mobility Day **Repeat 5 times** Any non impact cardio (bike, elliptical, row, swim) 5 minutes Foam roll or stretch 5 minutes **If pool available:** swim 5 minutes tread 5 minutes dynamic stretches in water 5 minutes If no pool do stretches in the Lower Back Plan	Cardio / Core 20 min bike Pyramid - each minute is tougher than previous minute. IF AVAILABLE 20 min walk/run combo on or just walk longer if you prefer. **Upper Core Spread throughout day:** **Repeat 2 times** Reverse pushups 10 Birds 10 Arm Haulers 10 Plank Pose 1 min	**Warmup with 10 min run or bike** **Repeat 5 times** Walk or walk/jog combo 5 minutes Pushups -___? Pullups - ____? or DB rows 10/arm Squats 10-15 Light weight shoulders *Cooldown cardio 15-20 minutes of walk, bike, jog..etc, Your choice for max distance.* Lower back plan – stretches Try to get an extra 40 minutes of cardio this weekend – spread throughout the weekend.

Week 8 – Calisthenics / Weights Progression – Cardio		
Day 1	Day 2	Day 3
Warmup with 5 minute cardio of choice

Lightweight Shoulder

Repeat 3 times
jumping jacks 10
squats 10
pushups 10
pullups 3

Repeat 3 times
Bench Press 10 or
Pushups 15
Crunches 1 min

Repeat 2-3 times
Pulldowns 10
DB rows 10
DB Thrusters 10
Rev crunches 1 min
Lunges 10/leg

Repeat 3 times
Squats 10
Double crunch 1min
MJDB#2 - 10
Plank pose 1 min

Lightweight Shoulder

Follow with steady cardio of walk, jog, bike, swim, elliptical or any of your choice for 20 min | Faster Paced Cardio options mixed with higher resistance:

Walk/jog combo - walk 1 min jog 30-60 seconds as long as you can

Or bike - fast /slow for 40-60 total minutes

Stop two times during the cardio section and do:

Core:
crunches 10
rev crunches 10
double crunches 10
left crunches 10
right crunches 10
bicycle crunches 10
plank pose 1 min
Rev pushups 10
Birds 10
Arm haulers 10

Lower back plan (stretches only) - do it later in the evening | Upper Body Plus Mobility Day

Repeat 5 times
jumping jacks 10
pushups 10
pullups 1-5

Repeat 5 times
bike, elliptical, row or swim 5 minutes
5 min stretch or foam roll

If pool
swim 5 min
tread water 5 min
dynamic stretches 5 min in chest deep water

OR

Follow with any cardio of your choice 10 minutes and dynamic / static stretches on land.

Repeat 2 times
Reverse pushups 10
Birds 10
Arm Haulers 10
Plank Pose 1 min |

Week 8 - Calisthenics / Weights Progression – Cardio		
Day 4	Day 5	Day 6
Faster Paced Cardio options mixed with higher resistance: Walk/jog combo - walk 1 min jog 30-60 seconds as long as you can **Or bike - fast /slow for 40-60 total minutes** Stop two times during the cardio section and do: Core: crunches 15 rev crunches 15 double crunches 15 left crunches 15 right crunches 15 bicycle crunches 15 plank pose 1 min Rev pushups 15 Birds 15 Arm haulers 15 Lower back plan (stretches only)- do it later in the evening	Push, Pull, Legs, Core **Lightweight Shoulder** **Repeat 2 times** 5 Min cardio Pushups 10-15 Pullups max DB rows 10 MJDB#2 - 10 reps **Repeat 2 times** 5 Min cardio Military press 15 DB bicep curls 10 DB squats 15 DB lunges 10 **Repeat 2 times** plank pose 1 min Pushups max crunches 25 Woodchopper squats 10 **Walk, jog, swim, or bike 10 minutes for max distance**	Faster Paced Cardio options mixed with higher resistance: Walk/jog combo - walk 1 min jog 30-60 seconds as long as you can **Or bike - fast /slow for 40-60 total minutes** Stop two times during the cardio section and do: Core: crunches 20 rev crunches 20 double crunches 20 left crunches 20 right crunches 20 bicycle crunches 20 plank pose 1 min Rev pushups 20 Birds 20 Arm haulers 20 Lower back plan (stretches only) - do it later in the evening

Week 9 - Calisthenics / Weights Progression – Cardio		
Day 1	Day 2	Day 3
Repeat 5 times Jumping jacks 10 Pushups 5-10 Plank pose 10 seconds **Repeat 2-3 times** Bench press 10 or Pushups max Pullups - max reps or DB rows 10 **Dips** - max MJDB#1 - 10 reps **Core Set:** crunches 15 rev crunches 15 double crunches 15 left crunch 15 right crunch 15 bicycle crunch 15 Reverse pushups 20 Birds 20 Arm haulers 20 Plank pose 1 min Lightweight Shoulders **Cardio Section:** 2 mile walk/jog mix OR row 10-20 min worth	5:00 warmup **Cardio / Leg Day Option:** Walk and/or jog mix 2 miles - every 5 minutes stop and do 20 squats or 10 lunges per leg. Bike, elliptical, row, or swim 20 min or walk 20 minutes Finish with Lowerback plan stretches only	Mobility Day **Repeat 5 times** Any non impact cardio (bike, elliptical, row, swim) 5 minutes Foam roll or stretch 5 minutes **If pool available:** swim 5 minutes tread 5 minutes dynamic stretches in water 5 minutes If no pool do stretches in the Lower Back Plan

Week 9 - Calisthenics / Weights Progression – Cardio		
Day 4	Day 5	Day 6
Repeat 3 times jumping jacks 10 pushups 10 squats 10 stretch **Push Set x 2:** Bench press 10-15 or Pushups 10-15 DB tricep ext. 10 Dips - 10-15 Lightweight Shoulders **Pull Set x 2:** Pullups - max Pulldowns 10 DB rows 10 DB bicep curls 10 DB Rows 10/arm MJDB#2 - 10 reps **Leg Set x 2:** Squats 20 Lunges 10/leg WC Squats - 10 MJDB#2 - 10 Cardio option of choice 20 minutes	5:00 warmup **Cardio / Leg Day** Walk and/or jog mix 2 miles OR row 1000m Or Bike / elliptical or swim 20 minutes BUT - every 5 minutes stop and do 20 squats or 10 lunges per leg. PLUS CORE SET from Day 1 Finish with Lower Back plan - stretches only	Warmup 5 minutes Full Body Day **Repeat 5 times** Jumping jacks 10 Pushups 10 Plank pose 30sec. Squats 10 Pullups 1-5 **Repeat 3 times** Bench Press 10 Pulldowns 10 Thrusters 10 Abs of choice 20 **Repeat 2 times** DB rows 10 Lunges 10/leg Farmer walks up/down stairs 3x Cardio option of choice 20 minutes

Week 10 - Calisthenics / Weights Progression – Cardio		
Day 1	Day 2	Day 3
Warmup with 5 min cardio option of your choice - jog, walk, bike, elliptical, rower. **repeat 3 times** Jumping jacks 10 Pushups 10 Birds 10 **Repeat 3 times** Cardio 5 min Bench press 10 Pullups max Db rows 10/arm Pushups – max Abs of choice 25 Plank pose 1 min **Do 1-2 times throughout workout** Lightweight shoulders 5# MJDB#1 - 10 Cardio Interval: 1 min fast - 1 min slow for 20 minutes **PT Reset** Reverse pushups 20 Birds 20 Arm haulers 20 Plank pose 1 min	**Cardio / Leg Day** Add in squats 10-20 reps every 10 minutes of cardio time 40-60 minutes of your choice: swim, bike, row, elliptical, jog... or mix 2 x 30 min options or 2-3 x 20 min options of above or others. can you push to 75-90 minutes of cardio???	Mobility Day **Repeat 5 times** Any non impact cardio (bike, elliptical, row, swim) 5 minutes Foam roll or stretch 5 minutes **If pool available:** swim 5 minutes tread 5 minutes dynamic stretches in water 5 minutes If no pool do stretches in the Lower Back Plan

Week 10 - Calisthenics / Weights Progression – Cardio		
Day 4	Day 5	Day 6
Calisthenics / Weights / Cardio Warmup with **Repeat 5 times** jumping jacks 10 Pushups 10 Reverse Pushups 10 **Repeat 3 times** Pullups max DB rows 10 Bench press 10 Plank pose 1 min Pullups max or Pulldowns 10 Pushups max Crunches 20 MJDB#1 - 10 Lightweight Shoulders Run 2 miles - for time-_____? or bike / elliptical / swim / rows 20 minutes	Cardio of your choice 60 minutes Note how far you get after 1 hour of walking, walking / running mix, backpacking, swimming, rowing, biking, or elliptical - your choice Divide 60 min through the day if you must..30 min in the am / pm	Warmup with 5 minute cardio of choice **Repeat 3 times** Bench press 10-15 Crunches 1 min Pulldowns 10-15 Rev crunches 1 min **repeat 2-3 times** Squats 10-15 Double crunch 1min MJDB#2 - 10 DB Thrusters 10 Pick an upper body push, pull, leg, and full body exercise and complete the circuit 3 times resting with abs after each exercise Follow with steady cardio of walk, jog, bike, swim, elliptical or any of your choice for 20-30 min

Week 11 - Calisthenics / Weights Progression – Cardio		
Day 1	Day 2	Day 3
Warmup with 5 min cardio option of your choice - jog, walk, bike, elliptical, rower...	Core / Cardio	Warmup With Non impact Cardio 5 min
	Cardio / Core x 2	
Repeat 5 times	Crunches - 20	**Squat Pyramid** - 1-
Jumping Jacks 10	Cardio 2 minutes	10 - run 25m 1 squat,
Pushups 5-10	Rev crunch 20	run 25m 2 squats,
	Cardio 2 minutes	run 25m 3...keep
Repeat 3 times	Double crunch 10	going to 10.
Bench press 10	toe touches - 10	
Military press 10	Left crunches - 20	5 min bike or
Tricep ext 10	Cardio 2 minutes	elliptical or rower
Pullups max and/or	Right crunches 20	
Pulldowns 10	cardio 2 minutes	**Repeat 3 times**
Bicep curls 10	Bicycle crunch 10	5 min tabata interval
	cardio 2 minutes	(20 sec sprint / 10
Repeat 3 times	plank pose 1 min	sec easy) on bike
MJDB#1 - 10		Squats 10
Dips 10	Lower back plan -	Lunges 10/leg no
DB rows 10/arm	do stretches and	weight
Crunches 25	core exercises	Farmer walk
Plank pose 1 min		up/down stairs 2x
Pushups Pyramid - 1-		Burn 100 calories
10 - run 25m 1 pushups,		burnout - how quickly
run 25m 2 pushups, run		can you burn 100
25m 3...keep going to		cals on any cardio
10.		machine? _____ or
		how fast can you
Cardio cooldown		run/walk 1 mile
10 min or more of your		
choice. Easy pace.		stretch legs

Week 11 - Calisthenics / Weights Progression – Cardio		
Day 4	Day 5	Day 6
Mobility Day **Repeat 5 times** Any non impact cardio (bike, elliptical, row, swim) 5 minutes Foam roll or stretch 5 minutes **If pool available:** swim 5 minutes tread 5 minutes dynamic stretches in water 5 minutes If no pool do stretches in the Lower Back Plan	**Fullbody** **Repeat 3 times** Cardio 5 min Squats 10-20 Bench press - 10 pullups max OR pulldowns 10,10 (wide, regular grip) crunches 20 Burpee or pushup pyramid 1-5: 1 pushup run 25, 2 pushups run 25 ...to 5 reps (or burpees) Lightweight shoulders **Repeat 3 times** MJDB#2 - 10 DB Rows 10/arm Thrusters – 5-10 Lunges 5/leg crunches 20 **Walk / jog 2 miles** or bike, row, swim 20 min	Core / Cardio **Cardio / Ab workout x 2** Crunches - 20 Cardio 2 minutes Rev crunch 20 Cardio 2 minutes Double crunch 10 toe touches - 10 Left crunches - 20 Cardio 2 minutes Right crunches 20 cardio 2 minutes Bicycle crunch 10 cardio 2 minutes plank pose 1 min Lower back plan - do stretches and core exercises WEEKEND GOAL Long weekend cardio of your choice - 60 minutes total swim, bike, row, elliptical, jog...or mix 2 x 30 min options or 3 x 20 min options of above or others.

Week 12 - Calisthenics / Weights Progression – Cardio		
Day 1	Day 2	Day 3
<u>Light weight shoulders</u>	5:00 warm up stretch	<u>Light weight shoulders</u>
Repeat 5 times jumping jacks 10 pushups - 10	**Cardio / Legs / Core** Walk, bike, swim, elliptical - get 30 minutes of either or mix of two or more for more than 30 minutes.	**Repeat 3 times** jumping jacks 10 pushups - 10
Repeat 3 times Bench press 10-20 Pullups max Pulldowns 10		**Repeat 3 times** Bench press 10-20 Pullups max Pulldowns 10
Repeat 3 times Pushups 10 Crunches 20 Reverse pushups 10 Birds 10 Arm Haulers 10 Plank Pose 1 min MJDB#1 - 10	BUT every 10 minutes stop and do Squats 20 Lunges 10/leg Plank pose 1 min	**Repeat 3 times** Pushups 10 Bicep Curls 10 DB rows 10 MJDB#1 - 10
Cardio Workout Tread or Swim 15-20 minutes or bike pyramid, elliptical or row Tabatas (20 sec fast / 10 sec slow for 15 minutes		**Lift / Core Cycle x1** Crunches 20 Pulldowns 10 Rev Crunches 20 Military press 10 Double crunch 10 MJDB#1 - 10 Left Crunch 20 DB rows 10/arm Right crunch 20 Cardio of choice 20 minutes

Week 12 - Calisthenics / Weights Progression – Cardio		
Day 4	Day 5	Day 6
Mobility Day **Repeat 5 times** Any non impact cardio (bike, elliptical, row, swim) 5 minutes Foam roll or stretch 5 minutes **If pool available:** swim 5 minutes tread 5 minutes dynamic stretches in water 5 minutes If no pool do stretches in the Lower Back Plan	5:00 warm up stretch **Cardio / Legs** Walk, bike, swim, elliptical - get 30 minutes of either or mix of two or more for more than 30 minutes. BUT every 10 minutes stop and do Squats 20 Lunges 10/leg Plank pose 1 min	Warmup with 5 min cardio of choice **Repeat 2 times** Bench press 10 Pulldowns 10 **Repeat 2 times** DB Rows 10/arm DB Thrusters 10 **Repeat 2 times** MJDB#1 - 10 Lightweight shoulder **Crunch Cycle x1** Crunches 20 Pulldowns 10 Rev Crunches 20 Military press 10 Double crunch 10 MJDB#1 - 10 Left Crunch 20 DB rows 10/arm Right crunch 20 **Weekend goal:** Walk 10-15 minutes after every meal or get in a 6th workout - Repeat any of the days of this week.

Lose the Body Fat / Inches

Going from highly active job with required morning workouts, bi-annual fitness tests, to retirement or a desk job can often lead to a quick and steady weight gain if you do not either continue the physical activity during retirement or learn how to eat like a person who does significantly less activity. Far too many people who change jobs or retire seem to forget how active they were prior to retirement and still eat like a highly active person. It does not take long for this error to yield a twenty-pound weight gain. This can happen in as little as a year, in fact, it often does. So, I think the first goal when you make a drastic change to your activity level is to make sure you tackle the food intake immediately. It is more and more difficult to out-work your diet, in fact, when of military retirement age it is nearly impossible. So, you have to hit your healthy weight and fitness from both ends: Calories IN and Calories OUT.

Ideas for the Calories IN Side of the Equation:

Make a list of EVERYTHING – Everything you eat, snack, drink all day long needs to be put on paper so you can see it and do the math. Add up the calories / portion sizes of every meal, snack, and drink. Also keep track of water intake. In fact, add more water (typically). PERSONAL CATCH: This was life changing. I realized I like to get a spoonful of peanut butter as a snack throughout the day. This is not an "unhealthy" snack, but does add up with calories. A few days a week, I added 800 calories to my day with a few spoons just because it was there. This adds up by the end of the week and was my main contributor maintaining / slowing gaining a pound a month. No more peanut butter in the house and I dropped five pounds in 2 weeks!

Be Smart – There are many Weight Loss Myths out there that many have tried with mixed short term but horrible long-term results. If you are starting to gain weight, avoid these myths.

Eat Smart – Think about what goes into your body. It does not take advanced education to realize the Ho-Ho's and soda are going to wreck your calorie intake and provide very little nutrients.

Eating plan - This eating plan will help your body keep the metabolism high and burn calories throughout the day. Limiting calories of processed sugar and other processed foods, adding fiber, and adding protein will help lean you out quickly and in a healthy manner.

Some Foods Should be Avoided and All Need to be Controlled – At increasing ages like ourselves, outworking your diet is a thing in the past. Your ability to consume more calories is easier but the ability to burn them off at higher rates is more difficult. I have found that it came down to more *portion control* for me than what I was eating. I do not eat sugar snacks, drink sodas, or sugary drinks, however, I will eat a second portion of chicken, steak, fish, peanut butter, and other nuts. These are high calories foods that are great for the body but controlling that urge to eat more has been the ticket to not gaining five pounds a year. If still hungry after dinner, and there is still more food just sitting there, save it for tomorrow. Try to top it off with a salad or extra glass of water.

Make a Plan of what you eat each week will keep the discipline in your world that you may even miss in retirement. After all, it is easy to work out for an hour a day, keeping poor food choices out of your mouth the other 23 hours requires the real motivation and discipline.

Get Out and Move to Get the Calories OUT:

The other half of the fitness and health equation is to keep moving. This can be a large variety of movements and activities.

Keep up your activity – If you are lucky to be this active and enjoy exercising as a daily habit. Keep this up, but play around with new training ideas and figure out roughly how many calories you are burning in a workout session. You can also add in your other outdoor activities like walking a dog, yard work, or other active hobbies too.

You may need to up your game a bit and add a second activity session into your day. If you are an early bird exerciser, that is great with a higher metabolism in the morning, but you may find that afternoons are sluggish. Especially, if you eat a big lunch followed by little activity. Now, a quick walk /jog of the dogs, a swim for 20 minutes, or bike ride helps after a smaller meal to stay awake and productive at work and burning more calories in the day

Exercise – Keeping a daily PT program in retirement is a must, but it does not have to be anything you use to hate about the military PT testing or standards. Some people like to "be all you can be" and still keep up with the Army PT Standards of running, pushups, situps. I would recommend replacing situps with plank poses for a better core activity, but other calisthenics like pushups, dips, pullups are great additions to any PT program and can be easily done at home.

Some form of cardio – Maybe by now, daily running has taken its toll on your knees or back. Perhaps replacing running with bike, elliptical, or rowing machines or swimming will be something to ride into retirement. If you still like to run, consider running every OTHER day and mixing in a non-impact options as above on the days in between running.

Non-Impact Cardio workouts - 4-5 times a week of 45-60 minutes of cardio exercises -elliptical gliding, walking, jogging, swimming, rowing, or biking are great examples of how to burn calories. If you are overweight and need to lose over 50 lbs I do not recommend running. Select a non-impact form of the aerobics listed above.

Stay Limber – If you sit too long during the day, you will start to ache. Get up and stretch. Check out the Lower back Plan for starters to stay limber and keep the core tight. But, consider yoga or other stretching and mobility programs to keep the joints working at full range of motion.

Get out of the house – Get to the gym and have access to pools, equipment, other fitness focused people. Play sports like Pickleball, racquetball, tennis if you are into competition on moderate to low levels of challenge. Get hardcore if you wish and try weight lifting contests or races if your joints can still handle it. The point is, have fun with your fitness and make it a way to be a social outlet as well.

See Links: Nutrition | ABDs of Nutrition | Lean Down

Gaining weight later in life (40 years and over) can be as easy as looking at food for most of us. Losing it however is much tougher than it was in our twenties. Men and women both have a decrease in metabolism after forty years old – some even earlier. We can however, fight the effects of aging with a steady AND daily exercise plan, stretching, de-stressing, and eating foods that are rich in protein, carbs, fats, vitamins, and minerals.

In closing, find out where the leaks are in your diet by keeping track of food coming in and see if you can add something to your exercise plan that burns more calories (higher intensity, duration, resistance training, etc). Avoid sugar and focus on foods that keep you full that are higher in fiber, vitamin rich nutrients as listed in the links above. Good luck. Time to get to work!

Open Invitation - FREE Workouts!

We do local training for FREE in the Annapolis / Severna Park MD area year-round. Our weekly schedule can be found at the Heroes of Tomorrow page. Check in with us prior to attending and fill out the questionnaire on the page above.

If you find this book helpful, let others know. You can also purchase multiple copies at a reduced price from our printer service if you have a large group of people who would benefit from this information. For any info on bulk purchases contact us at the email listed below for price savings per multi-book purchase.

ONLINE COACHING

Also, if you need personal training help, check out the StewSmithFitness.com website where you can train with me through the Online Coaching program.

GOOD LUCK

Thanks for choosing a profession of serving your country and community. It is an honorable profession that requires commitment to stay fit and healthy so you can best perform your duties, to stay alive, and keep others alive.

Good luck with the program and remember to consult your physician first before starting any program if you have not exercised in several months or years. If you need help with any fitness related questions please feel free to email me.

Contact us at stew@stewsmith.com if you need to ask questions about training, this specific workout, or you would like to attend our local workouts, make bulk purchases, or considering online coaching.

79917986R00052